MARTINA SCHOLZ
CLARISSA VON REINHARDT

STRESS IN DOGS

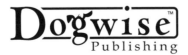

Wenatchee, Washington U.S.A.

Stress in Dogs
Martina Scholz and Clarissa von Reinhardt
Published by Dogwise Publishing
A Division of Direct Book Service, Inc.
PO Box 2778
701B Poplar
Wenatchee, Washington 98807
1-509-663-9115, 1-800-776-2665
website: www.dogwisepublishing.com
email: info@dogwisepublshing.com

ISBN: 1-929242-33-6

Printed in the U.S.A.

Library of Congress Cataloging-in-Publication Data
Scholz, Martina.
 [Stress bei Hunden. English]
 Stress in dogs / Martina Scholz, Clarissa von Reinhardt.
    p. cm.
 Includes bibliographical references and index.
 ISBN 1-929242-33-6
 1. Dogs--Behavior. 2. Dogs--Physiology. 3. Stress (Physiology) I. Reinhardt, Clarissa von. II. Title.
 SF433.S37 2007
 636.7'089698--dc22
                          2006030195

CONTENTS

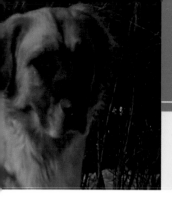

FOREWORD

Dear Reader,

You are now holding something precious in your hands, a detailed work on stress in our pet dogs, the like of which I have yet to find anywhere else.

The authors draw on many years of experience in training dogs. Due to their comprehensive knowledge of dogs - and of stress in particular - they have managed to present both the physiological and the psychological aspects of this subject in a reader-friendly manner. They have compiled a carefully composed list of stress factors indicating the experiences that might more or less seriously influence your dog. Although each individual factor in itself may probably only have a small effect, should more of these stress factors combine, it may endanger your dog's health and mental well-being.

Additionally, this book will improve your understanding of various stress symptoms – an important overview enhancing your ability to analyze your dog's behavior. Many, if not all, behavioral problems are more or less stress-induced. If you know that particular behavior is stress-related, it will be easier for you to find the stressors. And once you have found them, this book will provide you with ideas to create an anti-stress program that you can follow!

At the same time, the authors have also managed to explain the scientific aspects in such a way that even complex connections become clear. This makes it easy to work with this book actively. Additionally, if a dog is suffering from stress, numerous examples from daily training practice help you to understand what needs to be done and when, how and why you need to do it.

This book will give you many useful tips that will help you to better understand what is causing stress in your dog and what you can do about it. It is a treasure trove of experience – use it!

Anders Hallgren
Psychologist and animal behavior therapist

PUBLISHER'S NOTE
Dogwise Publishing is pleased to bring this book, originally published in Germany, on the topic of the physiology, recognition, and treatment of stress in dogs to the English language market. We believe that the reader will find the clear and concise examples and explanations of the common and uncommon signs of stress in dogs to be eye-opening and useful in their day-to-day interactions with dogs.

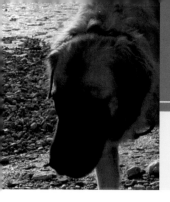

INTRODUCTION

The issue of stress has long been a vital part of human medicine and psychology. Scientific studies have proved that stress leads to health problems, affects our relationships with others and makes us unbalanced, irritable and aggressive towards our surroundings.

However, life in our highly technological, heavily de-naturized civilization does not only stress we humans, but also our dogs. The conditions under which dogs are kept today demand a lot from them. They are expected to deal with traffic and immense levels of noise. Dogs, despite their need for the company of other animals, are supposed to stay at home on their own for hours and then shine with good social behavior towards all other dogs and humans during a walk in the park. We want to be able to take them practically everywhere, regardless of whether it's to a shopping center, to a restaurant or into the middle of a crowded subway train. They are supposed to accompany us on forest walks, yet not show the slightest interest in wildlife. And so on...

Increasing regulations and legislation do not make things easier for our dogs either. In some federal states in Germany it is hardly possible anymore to let them romp and run around to their hearts' content, because the regulations for keeping dogs on leash make it impossible for their owner to give them more than a few yards of space. We humans are advised to let off steam by going jogging or doing other sports activities when we feel our stress levels rise. What about our dogs? Only a lucky few have a huge yard in which to run around.

As if this weren't enough, most dogs have to deal with con-siderably increasing hostility around them. If you become the target of verbal abuse during a walk, the dog will also sense a heightened degree of tension and will certainly not remain unaffected. Owners of big black dogs or the so-called fighting dog breeds (or whatever some people may consid-er fighting dogs...) in particular notice increasingly often that not only they, but also their dogs arrive home after each walk stressed out rather than refreshed and happy.

To assume that all of this does not have any impact on our dogs would be unrealistic. If you look at their lives, you can indeed find many reasons to support the theory that they could be stressed. Even if every organism can easily com-pensate for a certain level of stress, the time has come to consider whether our pet dogs have not long since exceed-ed this level.

When it comes to our four-legged companions, the impact of stress has long been underestimated. We have only seri-ously started to think in the last few years about how much stress a dog can actually bear before over-reactions or health problems occur, and so far there has been hardly any research into stress in dogs and other pets.

But what can be done? Get rid of all dogs because we have turned them into nothing more than stressed-out nervous wrecks that we don't want to do with? Absolutely not!

Dealing with the subject consciously is the first step towards change. If we recognize when and why our dog is stressed, we can defuse conflict situations or prevent them from oc-curring in the first place. This is what we want to accomplish-with this book.

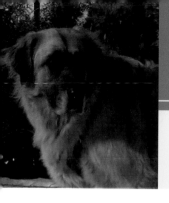

DEFINITION OF THE TERM STRESS

When dealing with the subject, you first have to define what stress actually is. The medical encyclopedia *Pschyrembel* contains the following definition:

"Stress (pressure, strain, tension) means a state of the organism which is defined by a specific syndrome (increased activity of the sympathetic nervous system, increased release of catecholamines, increased blood pressure, etc.), yet can be caused by various non-specific stimuli (infections, injuries, burns, radiation exposure, but also by anger, joy, pressure to perform and other stress factors). Stress can also mean the exogenous influences themselves to which the body is not sufficiently adapted. Psychological stress is a consequence of the discrepancy between specific demands and subjective coping. Continuous stress can lead to general reactions in terms of a general adaptation syndrome."

This means stress is a general term for numerous individual phenomena which are defined by a state of increased activity in the organism. In a neutral sense, stress means the organism's non-specific adaptation to any demand, i.e., an adaptive function. Most definitions describe stress as a state in which the organism reacts to an endogenous or exogenous (interior/exterior) threat and focuses its energies on coping with the situation of danger. Stress has always existed and, from an evolutionary point of view, it can be seen as a vital reaction to stimuli which has also enabled adaptation to changes in environmental conditions.

> ### WHAT IS STRESS?
>
> Most definitions describe stress as a state in which an organism reacts to an endogenous or exogenous threat and focuses its energies on coping with a dangerous situation.

At the same time, stress describes an ambivalent phenomenon for which the stress researcher Hans Seyle introduced the terms Eustress and Distress. Eustress is a necessary activation of the organism allowing the animal (or the human) to use its energies optimally and thus also enabling the development of capabilities. Distress, on the other hand means a damaging excess burden on the organism. During the past few decades, stress has predominantly been connected with a reduction in well-being, efficiency and health. In other words: references to stress practically always mean distress.

STRESS SHOWS ITSELF IN EVERY LEVEL OF THE ORGANISM:

- Physiologically, for instance in outbreaks of sweating, palpitations, etc.
- In behavior, for instance through aggression, agitation or restlessness.
- In perception, for instance in judging one's own state.

It can manifest itself in every aspect of life, in every situation and also at every age. The perception of stress as well as the coping strategies developed by the organism can be different from human to human and also among dogs. For example, different dogs experiencing the same situation perceive it differently, some not seeing it as stressful at all while others are clearly stressed by it. Completely different symptoms and coping strategies can be seen among those that show stress reactions.

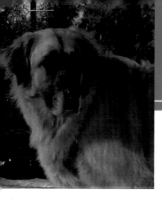

In situation-specific concepts of stress research, the focus lies predominantly on the releasing stimuli, the so-called stressors.

We differentiate between:

- Exogenous stressors such as flooding (overloading with stimuli) of the sensory organs or withdrawal of stimuli (deprivation), pain and real or artificially created states of danger.

- Withdrawal of food, water, sleep or physical exercise, so that primary needs cannot be satisfied anymore.

- Performance stressors, for example overburdening, lack of challenges, upcoming exams, possible failure, scolding or punishment.

- Social stressors through the dog's permanent exclusion from our life, such as isolation.

- Predominantly psychological stressors such as conflicts, lack of control, fear and insecurity about what to expect.

Major changes in circumstances such as the death of a person well known to the dog or changing residences can be perceived as stressors just as much as minor daily events piling up.

The reaction to stress can be sub-divided into three subsequent stages:

- **Stage one - the alarm reaction stage**
  In this stage, the interaction of nervous impulses and hormone release leads to optimum efficiency.

- **Stage two - the resistance stage**
  During this second stage, resistance towards the releasing factor is increased while resistance towards other stimuli is reduced. This means that the attempt to cope with the situation lowers resistance towards other stressors.

- **Stage three - the exhaustion stage**
  If the stress persists, the organism can no longer cope, despite the original adaptation. The symptoms of the alarm reaction from stage one reappear, but now they are permanent. This constant high tension can, in combination with other risk factors, lead to organic diseases and in extreme cases even to death.

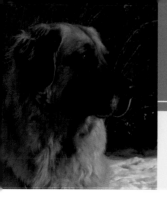

PHYSIOLOGY OF STRESS

WHAT HAPPENS INSIDE THE BODY WHEN WE ARE PUT UNDER STRESS?

As soon as the body is placed under stress, various hormones (summed up under the term "stress hormones") are released. These hormones alter numerous physical functions. In order to understand these alterations better, it is necessary to look at the normal state first. To maintain the normal state - the so-called homeostasis - the body has various circuits with negative feedback. This means: as soon as any hormone is released and its concentration in the blood has reached a certain level, this hormone at the same time inhibits the very factors that stimulate its release. In other words, from a certain concentration onwards, the hormone inhibits its own production. In this way, under normal circumstances it ensures that the hormone concentration in the blood is regulated at a constant level.

The hormone cortisol is increasingly released under stress. It is under the control of the hypothalamus, a part of the diencephalon ("interbrain"). It regulates many important bodily functions such as regulation of warmth, the wake-sleep pattern, regulation of blood pressure and respiration, control of food intake, of fat metabolism, and water balance.

In the hypothalamus, transmitters (so-called hypothalamic hormones) are produced and, if necessary, released. One of those hormones is the **C**orticotropin-**R**eleasing **H**ormone (**CRH**). The CRH released by the hypothalamus is transmitted directly to the pituitary gland, also called the hypophysis.

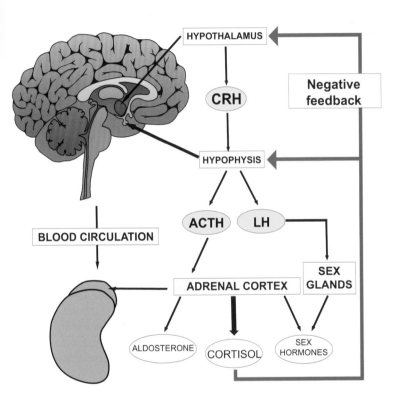

In the hypophysis, another transmitter, **A**dreno**c**orti**cot**ropic **H**ormone (**ACTH**), is released into the circulation. Through the blood, ACTH reaches the adrenal cortex where it stimulates, among other things, the release of cortisol.

The increased cortisol production leads to the above-mentioned negative feedback process due to the released cortisol inhibiting further production of ACTH and thus the further release of cortisol.

This is important in order to prevent an over-production of cortisol inside the body (see Figure 1).

Figure 1:
The negative
feedback process
seen through
the example
of cortisol.

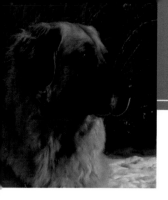

Cortisol belongs to the group of glucocorticoids that cause increased concentration of glucose (hence the name glucocortoids), amino acids, free fatty acids and urine in the blood. In this way all body cells are provided with more energy. At the same time, cortisol affects the immune system through inhibiting protein synthesis (building of protein) in the lymphocytes, resulting in a reduced number of defense cells. The best known characteristic of cortisol is its inhibitory effect on inflammation, by blocking inflammatory transmitters, the so-called cytokines.

In addition to cortisol, the adrenal cortex produces other hormones. Due to its regulating role of the minerals potassium and sodium, aldosterone (which belongs to the mineralocorticoids) has an important function in the organism's water balance. Small amounts of anabolic sex hormones such as testosterone are also released by the adrenal cortex. Testosterone has an anabolic effect - that is, it builds muscles and it also influences the mental state. A higher concentration of testosterone, especially resulting from hormone production in male animals' testicles is, for instance, connected to a higher readiness for aggression, which is particularly prevalent in the animal world.

Stress alters the normal state of the body's feedback control system. The body's first response to stress, whether caused by emotional or great physical strain, is the release of adrenaline from the adrenal medulla. This is caused by stimulation of the sympathetic nervous system, a part of the autonomic nervous system. Activation of the sympathetic nervous system and the corresponding release of adrenaline occurs involuntarily and almost instantly. Surely every human knows the tickling sensation and the "rush of blood" through the veins brought on by a sudden scare. This results from the effect of the adrenaline. Adrenaline, a neurotransmitter be-

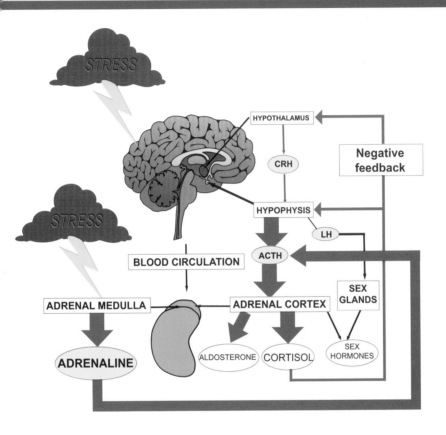

longing to the catecholamines, causes numerous alterations inside the body, such as a raised pulse and cardiovascular activity, increased systolic blood pressure and raised blood sugar, dilation of the bronchial tubes and of the pupils, as well as increased need for oxygen and a rise in free fatty acids in the blood.

Figure 2:
The effects of stress
on the feedback
control system.

Furthermore, adrenaline has an impact on the pituitary gland where it stimulates an increased release of the transmitter ACTH, and thus indirectly also on the adrenal cortex, which releases increasing amounts of stress hormones such as cortisol into the blood (see Figure 2).

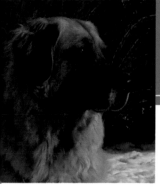

So, through the endocrine system (that is, through the hormone system) stress raises blood pressure and increases cardiovascular activity and heart rate. At the same time, the hormonal effect provides the body's cells with extra energy in the form of glucose and free fatty acids. In other words, stress at first leads to optimum efficiency. This can be seen as the biological purpose of stress, because in nature it is of vital importance for survival that the organism responds with optimum efficiency to a fright or heightened tension. This is the only way an individual can save its life by escaping, or how a predator can be successful at hunting. This type of stress can also be called positive stress or Eustress.

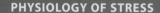

REACTIONS TO STRESS

At first, the body reacts to stress with exhaustion. If this is not followed by a long recovery phase, so-called adaptation diseases are to be expected.

Naturally, the body cannot keep up this state of alarm forever, and therefore negative phenomena will occur if the strong tension lasts for a longer period of time, or if situations of fright or shock frequently occur. At first, the body reacts to stress with exhaustion. If no long recovery phase follows, so-called adaptation diseases, such as kidney and cardiovascular diseases, are to be expected.

Cortisol is the main culprit for adaptation diseases. Normally, the half-life of cortisol is 20 minutes, i.e. , after 20 minutes the level of cortisol in the blood has dropped by 50%. Tests on animals have shown that under stress the negative feedback of the release of cortisol does not work anymore, and so within a few days, four times as much cortisol as normal is present. If the animal is in a situation that causes a permanent feeling of insecurity about what to expect and/or of helplessness, this effect is greatly reinforced. In human medicine it is assumed today that depression results among other things from exactly this effect.

However, dogs indeed often find themselves in exactly this situation of helplessness and insecurity about what to expect. For instance, dogs cannot estimate what will happen in situations humans control. Quite the opposite, we often behave inappropriately when we do not have the necessary expertise to grasp the situation. For instance, we make our dog feel helpless if a short leash, a head halter or similar device prevents him from reacting adequately to a situation. For example, the dog would like to create some distance between himself and another dog or walk in a curve, but is prevented from doing so.

More importantly, a permanently-raised level of cortisol in the blood weakens the immune system. Further consequences are diseases of the digestive system such as stomach ulcers and chronic diarrhea. In the long term it can lead to serious damage to the adrenal gland. Alterations of the cardiovascular and circulatory system such as high blood pressure, heart attacks, strokes and many other diseases can also result from long-term stress. Reproductive disorders

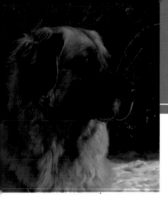

are connected to a permanently-raised level of cortisol. The maturing of ova in female animals as well as the production of testosterone and the development of spermatozoa in the male animal rely on a transmitter in the pituitary gland, the so-called luteinizing hormone (LH). Cortisol inhibits the release of LH and thus suppresses the maturing of ova or spermatozoa in the sex glands (ovaries in the female, testicles in the male animal). Problems with the breeding of animals held in captivity (e.g. in a zoo) are caused by this effect.

Aldosterone, which is also released by the adrenal cortex, can, in the long term, cause a shift in the body's mineral and water balance, which will also show in high blood pressure.

A certain amount of stress is sensible and – for optimum physical efficiency – even necessary. Up to a certain point every organism can compensate for stress without suffering damage. The question of where this point is depends on the extent of the stress suffered. If the body compensates for stress situations, i.e., if it gets accustomed to a certain level of stress, this is referred to as adaptation syndrome, or coping.

If this process of coping is not possible anymore, adaptation diseases as described above will occur, a situation referred to as Distress (see Figure 3).

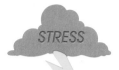

Eustress:
Optimum readiness to react
and physical efficiency through
increased energy supply
to the body

Distress:
Pathological alteration through
enduring or high stress, such as diseases
of the immune system, the kidneys,
the cardiovascular and circulation system
and the digestive system. Increased
readiness for aggression.

Figure 3:
Positive and nega-
tive consequences
of stress

In addition to various stress-induced diseases, Figure 3 also lists increased readiness for aggression as a possible consequence of stress. This is also related to the release of hormones, including the sex hormone testosterone. Recent studies in dogs show that, despite the increased release of cortisol, in specific stress situations testosterone levels are also raised.

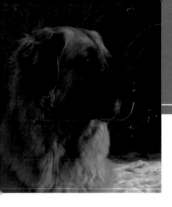

An illustration of the increased readiness for aggression due to testosterone can be observed in those species of animals whose mating season is limited to only a few weeks per year. Often the males gather one or more females around themselves and react particularly negatively and aggressively toward other males. They are constantly ready to defend their females against rivals. This behavior only occurs during the mating season and is closely linked to the naturally raised hormones levels at this time. This mechanism enables the males to get on reasonably well with each other outside of the mating season and prevents unnecessary conflict. This can be seen as a sensible link between sex hormones and readiness for aggression.

The situation is different in dogs. Male dogs are not limited to a specific mating season and react throughout the year to female dogs in season. If many female dogs live in their environment, it will often be the case that one of them is in season and, due to raised testosterone levels, the male dog will show a correspondingly increased readiness for aggression towards other male dogs.

Long-term stress or frequently repeated stress situations can, under certain circumstances, also lead to raised sex hormone levels in the blood and therefore to a lower aggressive behavior threshold. This does not mean that every stressed dog will always and immediately react in an aggressive manner. It can mean, however, that the dog will react more strongly than usual in certain situations and that he is no longer able to deal with previously unproblematic situations such as joggers, cyclists, or other dogs.

Permanently-raised testosterone due to stress and/or continuing encounters with female dogs in season will have an impact on the health of the male dog, potentially resulting in the disease prostatic hyperplasia. In contrast to humans, this will not show through a urethral stricture and therefore through problems with urinating. In the male dog, the enlarged prostate presses on the rectum, causing problems with defecation.

> **REACTIONS TO STRESS**
>
> If a dog needs to defecate soon after entering a training site, despite having just been for a long walk, the cause is often excitement and/or stress.

Other symptoms or behavior that can be seen in a dog are also directly linked to the effects of stress. For instance, the saying "I am soiling myself with fear" actually has a physiological background and applies to both humans and dogs. In the event of great anxiety or a sudden fright, the release of adrenaline and the activation of the sympathetic nervous system signal the rectum to defecate.

If a dog needs to defecate soon after entering the training site, despite having just been for a long walk, the cause is often excitement and/or stress. This could be referred to as the almost obligatory "training mess." It makes absolutely no sense to scold the dog or to even punish him because he "has got to go"! Warnings to the dog owners to not let their dogs "foul the site" typical of many dog schools - let alone the bad habit of demanding fines for the club funds - also seem absurd if you know the reason for this defecation. Under closer examination, the argument that other dogs on the training site would be distracted by the scent

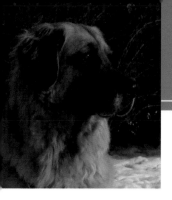

markings (whether through stools or urine) and would then be unable to concentrate properly on the commands is also absurd. For, after all, where can we go for walks with our dog without him being distracted by thousands of scent markings, and he (of course) still has to obey. Therefore, if your dog needs to defecate on the training site, please let him do so in peace and do not feel guilty about it. If you dispose of the remains afterwards, there are no problems with fouling the area either.

At dog shows you can often observe dogs struck by diarrhea, also mostly caused by stress. The confined space and the noise in the show rooms from masses of unknown people and other dogs is too much for many dogs. The continuing stress disturbs the water balance in such a way that diarrhea occurs.

REACTIONS TO STRESS
A male dog that constantly marks everywhere on the training site is not necessarily dominant, but might be seriously stressed.

If the dog is frequently put through such situations, chronic diarrhea will be the consequence. It is not a rare thing for the clueless dog owner to then consult numerous vets, try out all sorts of diets and remedies without achieving any satisfying results. No wonder, because the diarrhea is not caused by an infection of the digestive system, but by stress.

The bladder and kidneys are also influenced by stress hormones. Under stress, aldosterone is released and, together with adrenaline, stimulates kidney activity, resulting in increased urination. A male dog that constantly marks everywhere on the training site is not necessarily dominant, but might be seriously stressed.

Other situations that afflict the dog also show in an increased need to urinate. For example, the male Dalmatian Dandy does not often have to stay alone at home. However, when he does have to, he makes it very clear that he needs to go outside after his owner has returned – even though it is actually not yet time for the next walk. Finally outside, he stops at the nearest tree in order to relieve himself, taking noticeably longer than usual. The same happens to us humans. Whether taking a driving test or walking down the aisle, most of the time we go to the restroom shortly before.

Continuous stress can also cause bladder and kidney diseases. Permanent pressure on the bladder can lead to incontinence which means that the dog can no longer control and hold in the urine, and so soils himself. Kidney disease is also often caused (among other things) by permanent stress.

If a dog is often ill, suffers from allergies or catches practically every gastrointestinal virus that's going around you have to contemplate an immune system disorder. As already mentioned, cortisol released under stress can weaken the immune system.

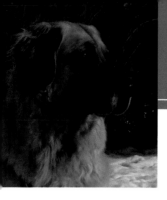

A constantly panting dog might also have a stress problem. Adrenaline accelerates circulation and respiration that, in addition to an increased pulse rate, also manifests itself in panting. If for instance a dog always pants during a car journey, you do not only have to check the inside temperature of the car but also whether the dog is generally afraid of being taken in a car and thus his panting is stress-induced.

IMPORTANT: The previously described examples of dogs having to deal with overburdening, fear or illness, are not the only causes of stress. Even situations we would consider to be positive, such as playing ball, can cause stress. Very positive, surprising experiences do not only excite humans, but also dogs.

Imagine someone informs you that you have won two million dollars on the lottery. Would you stay sitting and think, "Oh, that's nice?" Definitely not. You would shout out, be happy, your pulse rate would shoot up, you would be excited. Or think about a child who is having his or her birthday party. Many friends have been invited, there are presents galore,

Monday	Tuesday	Wednesday
Agility	Rambling in the mountains	Walk through the city center

relatives are coming to visit, games are being played. All day long this little person is the center of attention – and is correspondingly wound up, can't get to sleep at night, has to talk about all those experiences again and again until eventually he or she is able to calm down. Now imagine you celebrate this child's birthday every day for a week – he or she would never calm down again.

If you look at some dogs' "schedule," this is exactly what happens. Monday - agility with a group. Tuesday - walks in the mountains with six other dogs. Wednesday - walk through the city center including shopping in the shopping centers, followed by a meal in a restaurant. Thursday - obedience training in a mixed dog group. Friday - running alongside your bike to get his exercise. And now it's finally the weekend and we get to do some joint activities with our four-legged friend! All this is surely meant well, but it does not give the dog enough time to rest and yet again causes stress.

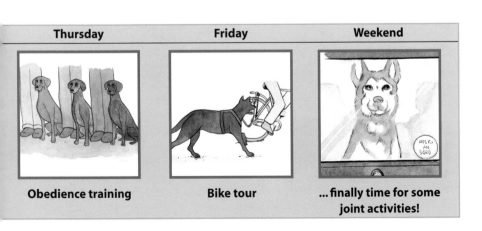

Thursday	Friday	Weekend
Obedience training	Bike tour	... finally time for some joint activities!

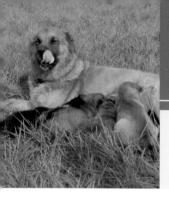

STRESS SYMPTOMS

Calming signals are often shown by a dog if he feels insecure, stressed or overburdened.

There are quite a few symptoms that indicate a dog might be stressed, and usually more than one of them occurs at the same time. Observe your dog, try to find out whether you can recognize one or more of such symptoms and what might be causing them.

IMPORTANT: Of course, some of these types of behavior also appear when the dog is not stressed, such as panting. He may only be panting because it is a really hot day, or because he has just played extensively. You must always consider the context for such behavior.

Another criterion is the question of how often the behavior occurs. If, after taking the whole picture into consideration, you get the impression that the behavior is actually stress-induced, you should think about changes. You will find ideas and inspiration for doing so in the chapter on the Anti-Stress Program.

A dog which seems harried and restless might be suffering from stress.

Nervousness
The dog is very easily startled, seems generally jumpy and nervous.

Restlessness
This may appear as constant fidgeting. The dog can only relax with difficulty or not at all, is unable to calm down even in the places where he usually lies down and pays a lot of attention to any noise. Often such dogs also pull hard on the

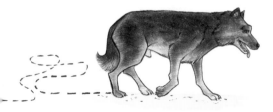

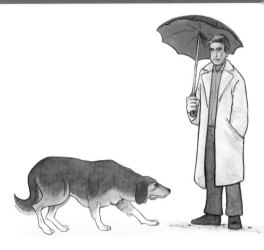

leash because they lunge forward as if they were being hunted.

Overreaction
The dog suddenly reacts in a restless, timid or aggressive manner to events or situations in which he would normally stay calm and relaxed.

Calming Signals
They are often shown by a dog if he feels insecure, stressed or overburdened.
If even the trained eye cannot notice any signals anymore, the dog might be so stressed that he has stopped this form of communication, perhaps even "freezes" (which means that he does nothing anymore).

A worsening of the situation is called "mental submergence". In her book *On Talking Terms With Dogs: Calming Signals* (Dogwise Publishing, 2006), Turid Rugaas illustrated the case of a Do Khyi which was so overburdened that he "became literally psychotic, withdrew from reality into an inner world where no bad things could reach him".

If a dog suddenly reacts in an unusual manner to situations which are actually familiar to him, it could be a sign of stress.

The processes inside the body under stress often make the dog defecate and urinate a number of times.

Defecation and urination
Both can be examples of stress symptoms. In the event of great fear or a sudden fright, the release of adrenaline and the activation of the sympathetic nervous system signal the rectum to defecate. Additionally, shifts in the water balance occur, resulting in a more frequent need to urinate.

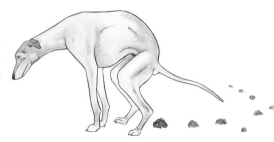

Unsheathing of the penis in male dogs

Usually only the front part - sometimes even only the tip - is unsheathed. Therefore this behavior can easily be distinguished from that of a sexually-stimulated male dog which is ready to breed.

Mounting

Mounting is not always sexually motivated but can also be stress-induced. It often occurs in mixed dog groups and is commonly mistaken as a gesture of dominance. However, leading cynologists agree that mounting, with its typical push movements of the pelvis, is not necessarily dominant behavior, unlike the T-position, biting the nose area and putting the head onto another dog's neck or back area.

Mounting is not always sexually-motivated but can also be stress-induced.

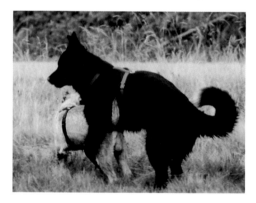

By the way, mounting not only occurs with other dogs, but also with humans or objects, such as the dog's own sleeping blanket or the sofa cushion. It is not only done by male dogs, but by female dogs as well.

If a puppy shows this kind of behavior, it can be a stress symptom, but it can also be just a playful way of trying out patterns of behavior without any serious intention behind it. In order to be able to decide on one of the two options, you have to look at the complete situation and it's greater context.

EXAMPLE: *At the age of only twelve weeks, a Golden Retriever showed this behavior every time there were visitors. After full-blown greeting ceremonies including extensive stroking and never-ending praise for this super-cute puppy, he was so beside himself that he either mounted the visitors or his blanket. After the visitors' greetings had dropped to a normal level, this behavior was no longer observed.*

Hypersexuality/ hyposexuality

Stress can lead to either an excessive libido or an almost complete loss of sexual drive. In this case dog owners either observe that their dog reacts in an overly-assertive manner to the opposite sex, or that their dog shows demonstrably little interest in potential sexual partners.

Altered sexual cycle

In female dogs, stress leads relatively often to alterations in the sexual cycle. The periods between the states in season are either too short or too long. Sometimes stress even has the effect that sexually-mature female dogs will not be in season for years. However, the so-called "continuous heat", where the female dog bleeds longer than usual and smells attractive to male dogs, can also be stress-induced.

Exaggerated self-grooming leading to wounds caused through licking is often a sign of – and at the same time compensation for – stress.

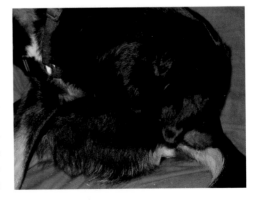

Exaggerated self-grooming

Can lead to self-inflicted wounds caused through licking, often at the extremities, at the tail and in the genital area. Should these parts of the body be so open and swollen that they are painful, the body releases endorphines (so-called "happy hormones") that ease the pain and lift the mood. This euphorigenic effect enables the dog to bear crippling situations more easily, and so a vicious circle is started that is difficult to break.

Destroying objects

This is often wrongly referred to as "destructive protest fury," especially if the dog shows this behavior when left alone. In fact, it is a sign of serious stress.

Exaggerated noise making

For example, continuous barking, permanent whining and howling are also often interpreted as protest behavior, but rather indicates that the dog is extremely overburdened and stressed.

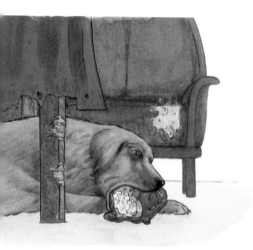

Disorders of the digestive system

Symptoms such as diarrhea and vomiting are among the most frequent and noticeable symptoms of stress. Some breeds are particularly prone, such as for example Collies, German Shepherds and Cavalier King Charles Spaniels.

To be left alone is so crippling to many dogs that they destroy objects and occasionally also the furniture.

Allergies

Allergic reactions to food, mites, flea bites, pollen, grass, insecticides, etc., can be stress-induced, or at least the course of the allergy can be quite considerably influenced by the dog's level of stress, for stress that continues over a longer period of time weakens the immune system due to the increased level of cortisol.

EXAMPLE: *The previously mentioned male Dalmatian who had a genetic allergy to food was, in the course of a training program, confronted with other male dogs to practice such encounters. However, since the training units were too long and took place too often and the dog had not enough time to recover, he at first reacted with spot-like skin rashes that eventually burst, leaving extensive inflammation with heavy dandruff - his allergy had literally exploded. After training had been reduced and the dog had longer resting periods, his state of health noticeably improved.*

Appetite loss

Everybody has heard of a dog that is so stressed he is unable to eat. It is a typical behavior when a dog is placed in a new environment, such as an unfamiliar boarding kennel or where he feels uncomfortable. When a dog is overburdened in training, he also spits out even the most delicious and otherwise much-loved treats or does not take them in the first place.

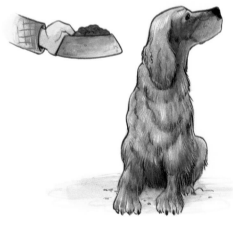

Over-eating

The dog frantically gulps down whatever he can find, unfortunately also inedible things such as paper tissues, stones, wood, etc. This behavior can be dangerous or even life-threatening in the event of an intestinal blockage, or of injuries to the digestive system caused by sharp objects. Caution! It is not enough to generally forbid the dog from taking such objects! The cause for the stress has to be found, or else the dog will find other ways to compensate.

A dog which does not want to eat even the most delicious food is often too stressed.

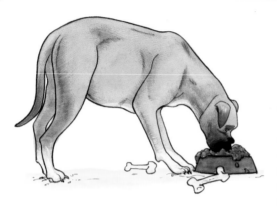

EXAMPLE: *When out for a walk, a female livestock guardian dog ate everything she found. In a dog school she was successfully trained not to take anything from the ground. The problem seemed to be solved and the owner was satisfied. Shortly after, the dog started to excessively lick and bite herself in the region around the base of the tail, as if she had fleas or the anal scent glands were full.*

The vet's examination didn't find anything wrong and nobody seemed to be able explain why she did what she did. Eventually, the woman changed dog schools and the new trainer found the cause of the behavior. The dog was stressed out by the tension at home between the owner and her partner due to the woman's decision to get a dog. There were constant arguments and the man made the dog fully aware that her presence was not appreciated. The dog soon started to swallow any objects she could find, as a type of compensation behavior. When this possibility was taken away from her, she showed a different type of compulsive behavior disorder leading to self-harming. It was made crystal clear to the owner that she had to choose between the man or the dog. The woman opted for the dog. Soon after they separated, peace had returned to the house and life had harmonized, the behavior completely disappeared.

If dogs indiscriminately gulp down everything edible or even indigestible, this over-eating is often caused by stress.

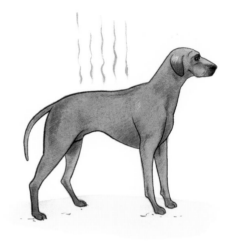

Unpleasant body odor and bad breath

Both can be caused by stress. Bad breath in particular is prevalent because the stressed dog pants more. In dogs as in humans, stress raises the secretion of gastrointestinal acids that then become noticeable through the unpleasant smell.

The dogs' whiskers

Whiskers become stiff and possibly even tremble. This is a symptom that can, by the way, also be observed in cats.

Raised hackles

Often wrongly interpreted as a sign of aggression, stiffening of the hairs on the back and neck occurs when the dog is stressed, feels insecure, is extremely happy and/or in other emotionally charged situations. In order to work out which particular emotion is involved, you need to take into account the complete situation and the rest of the dog's expressions. By way of example, when we are away from home too long, because she is so delighted to see us again, our female mongrel Elsa's hackles are so stiff that she looks like an upturned brush.

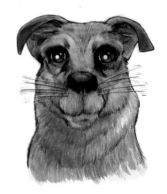

Unpleasant body odor, bad breath, and trembling whiskers are clear signs of stress.

Tense muscles due to increased muscle contraction
The main reason a stressed dog should never be forced to carry out "sit" and "down" commands is that it takes away the possibility for the dog to use movement to loosen and relax his tense muscles.

If the dog doesn't have the chance to move, it could result in trembling or even in painful muscle cramps, which then lead to greater readiness for aggression. In extreme cases, the cramps can be so strong that they resemble an epileptic fit.

For this reason movement is essential during situations of stress – in humans as well as in animals. You can observe this in yourself. When you're angry, you flap your arms, walk up and down, and gesture. Can you imagine yourself sitting calm and still while you are boiling with anger?

Dandruff
This is often associated with dry skin and can appear quite spontaneously. Dandruff is frequently observed in Dobermans and Rottweilers, but can also be seen in other breeds. During visits to the vet in particular, the dog practically flakes away.

Sudden moulting
This is often observed during dog exhibitions and shows. Claustrophobia, the noise levels, the inability to escape and the constant pulling and tugging can cause the dog's stress levels to shoot up. This is particularly noticeable in Dalmatians due to their white hairs sticking everywhere.

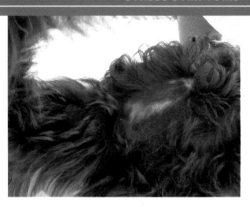

Bad coat condition and heavy moulting

Over a long period of time, both can be a symptom of stress. This can result in bald patches appearing in the coat.

Unhealthy appearance

The dog appears generally overburdened and sickly. Alongside the above-mentioned symptoms such as hair loss, dandruff and so on, the dog's eyes are dull and sunken, his posture is sagging and crouched, and his tail is hanging.

Sudden moulting – even with bald patches in the coat– sadly are classic stress symptoms.

Skin problems

Eczema, itchiness and open wounds are all classic stress symptoms.

Eye color changes

This is often seen during times of extreme stress but it is unclear why this happens. The eyes can also be blood-shot when high blood pressure causes the tiny blood vessels in the eye to burst.

Panting

Under stress the heart beat increases and the muscles tense, resulting in a greater need for oxygen. At the same time increased metabolic activity produces extra warmth. Panting supplies the body with more oxygen and additionally prevents the body from overheating.

A dripping nose

In some dogs, excitement and stress lead to increased nasal fluid production.

Sweaty paws

Although dogs do not have as many sweat glands as humans, they do have some, for example on the underside of the paws. A stressed dog sweats more, which can be observed in moist paw prints on smooth floors. This is especially prevalent in vets' waiting and examination rooms.

Trembling

As muscle contraction increases during stress, the body tries to loosen the tense muscles through movement in order to prevent cramps.

Frantic teeth snapping

This is a clear sign that the dog is stressed and it has all become too much for him. For example, where running around gets him too worked up or he feels cornered, he snaps around himself without biting his opponent. This deliberately off-target snapping is accompanied by clearly audible and visible snapping of the teeth.

Startled eyes / flickering gaze

Just as in humans, a dog's eyes open wide when he is frightened. Under extreme strain this can result in uncontrollable eye movements, described as a flickering gaze.

Staring intensely at another animal or object
The dog keeps the thing he finds stressful or scary firmly in view in order to assess what he believes the dangerous thing is going to do and be able to react accordingly with fight or flight.

Compulsive behavior
A distinction is made between compulsive movement and compulsive noise making. The behavior is kept up over a long time period and/or repeated in the same manner without there being an obvious reason for it. For example running in a figure of eight, running around in circles, chasing his own tail, monotonous barking and excessive licking are observed.

Biting the leash
For many dogs a sign of stress is when they start to bite the leash and to tug wildly on it. At first this behavior seems like a game but the dog is trying to work off stress. Observe your dog and try to see whether this behavior appears after situations that are tense and difficult for him to deal with.

EXAMPLE: *After exactly 20 minutes of obedience training a German Shepherd began to bite his leash and seemed to be unable to snap out of this behavior. After the owner noticed that the dog always displayed this behavior after the same amount of time, he simply stopped the training session five minutes earlier.*

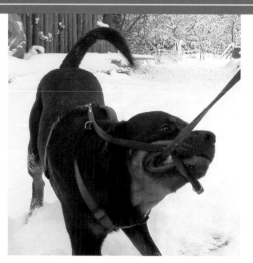

If a dog bites and tugs wildly on the leash, he is trying to work off and compensate for the stress he is under.

Other dogs display this behavior when they become stressed during a walk or when shopping trips get too much for them. Try to find out what sparks this behavior. If you think you have found the cause, stop doing it and wait and see if the leash biting goes away of its own accord.

This behavior is particularly prevalent in animal shelters. Living with other dogs at such close proximity places an enormous burden of stress on these dogs. It is also frequently not possible for all dogs to go for regular walks and the possibilities for running free are limited. The dog gets even more worked up when someone finally fetches him from the kennel to go for a walk. On top of his pent-up urge to move and the stress comes the excited anticipation of finally being able to run around – and off he goes again… You can imagine how much worse it must be for such a dog when he gets labelled a leash biter and is taken only reluctantly or not at all for walks. His frustration rockets and the problem worsens, sometimes to such an extent that the dog doesn't just bite the leash but also nips clothes or the walker. One possible solution involves not immediately putting the dog on the leash and then going for a walk but to speak to him calmly, possibly to offer him a treat and to wait until he is halfway settled. When you then take him out he will be still worked up – but less than before.

Poor concentration
The dog looks distracted and is unusually nervous during training. His concentration on new tasks and exercises is very poor.

Forgetfulness
The dog seems to have forgotten exercises he previously mastered. He looks as if he has had a black out. In normal everyday situations he seems to be "on another planet".

Re-directed behavior / displacement activity
The dog does something that does not seem appropriate for the situation. Often this type of behavior is a display of calming signals, which are in fact in some way connected to the situation.

If a dog acts in a way that does not seem appropriate, it is frequently a case of calming signals or re-directed behavior.

EXAMPLE:
Every time the female Giant Schnauzer Ginger met another dog, she sat down and started to scratch herself thoroughly. She did this until the other dog was close to her and friendly contact was established and possibly they had started to play together. If this game became too wild and hectic, she began to sniff the ground intensively. Her owner considered both types of behavior to be displacement activities. In fact, Ginger used them as calming signals that were understood by the other dog.

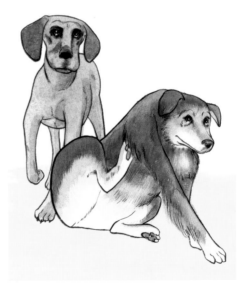

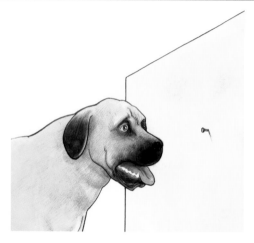

Staring intensely at something of no apparent interest is a stress symptom commonly seen in herding dogs.

Staring Intensely

Staring intensely at something interesting such as flies and light beams can be a sign of stress. The dog is unable to concentrate on anything else other than this captivating object and follows it – although sometimes only with the eyes – or chases after it, snapping at it and seems generally restless, agitated, and nervous.

Passivity

If you notice that your dog seems to be significantly quieter and more withdrawn than normal, then it could be a sign that your dog is overwhelmed by a situation he can't resolve.

EXAMPLE:

Into a household with a male Do Khyi and a small female mongrel came a five-year old female German Shepherd that the owner had found. In the following weeks the German Shepherd dominated the small female mongrel to such an extent that she hardly dared to leave her bed. She was noticeably quiet and had reduced her movements considerably, making every effort not to provoke the bigger, stronger German Shepherd. Although she actually had a lively, quirky personality and enjoyed barking when visitors arrived or it was time for a walk, it was almost *like she wasn't there anymore. The owner noticed this and, after all attempts to defuse the situation had failed, she decided to find a new home for the German Shepherd, which she succeeded in doing. After the bigger dog had moved in with friends, the small lady blossomed again. Even today, with 14 years of age, she jumps around and barks loudly when visitors come, just as she always has done.*

Shaking himself

Shaking is an indicator that a dog finds a situation exhausting. As soon as he recognizes that the situation is no longer threatening or is over, he releases tension by shaking himself.

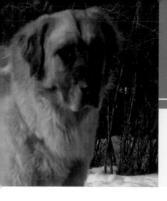

STRESS RELEASING FACTORS

Stress can also be looked at as a reaction by the organism to over-exertion, such as increased physical activity, warmth, cold, and external irritations or damage. Stress can also arise after sudden occurrences such as a fright or a shock. This over-exertion can arise from permanent or repetitive strains, however small, which do not allow the dog to rest and may lead to stress. The following list, by no means exhaustive, gives you several examples.

Disorders affecting the dog's functions
Such as lack of mobility or cardiovascular and kidney conditions, etc.

Disorders affecting the dog's senses
Such as deafness, blindness, limited sense of touch, etc. The dog does not have the same possibilities as a healthy dog to find its way around in the outside world and has to constantly compensate for deficiencies.

Disorders connected to temporary or chronic pain
Such as injuries, blood loss, infection, trauma, shock, rheumatoid arthritis, hip dysplasia, spondylosis, etc. Also worth mentioning is sensitivity to the weather, as difficult for dogs as for humans.

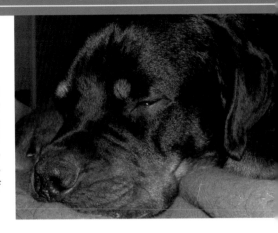

Hypersexuality
If we take the example of the male dog (where this is more prevalent than for the female), he is not the only one who is stressed due to his pent-up sexual drive. His overbearing behavior also stresses the other dog, which has the dubious honor of being the object of his desire.

Female dogs in season
This is a normal situation that also contains a number of stress factors, such as warding off overbearing males when she is not yet ready for copulation. Therefore, you should make the rest of her life as trouble-free as possible.

Lack of sleep can also occur when the dog does not have sufficient places to withdraw.

Lack of sleep
This can occur through illness and pain or when the dog does not have sufficient places to withdraw to or when his need for rest is not respected.

State of exhaustion
This can arise not only from lack of sleep but also from over-exertion during walks, dog sports or games.

Sudden changes
Such as moving home, an addition to the family, a new owner, etc.

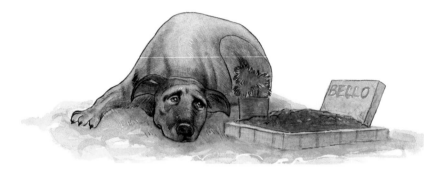

Dogs also feel grief when the person they were close to or a playmate dies.

Grief due to the loss of a partner

Dogs do not only grieve for the person they were close to but also for other animals they lived with or for playmates they met on daily walks. The degree and duration of the grief depends on how strong the bond was.

Threat

This can be real or imaginary. The dog may not able to logically distinguish between a real threat or one he feels is there, despite there actually being no danger present. In both cases his body goes into a state of alarm.

Expectations anxiety

The dog doesn't know what is being expected of him or cannot assess the situation. For example, he is expected to follow commands during an exercise he doesn't understand.

Imagine you are in a foreign country and you ask for directions to the restroom. A local helpfully gives you the necessary information but in a language you either don't or only partially understand. You try your best but his explanations are too difficult to follow. After a number of unsuccessful at-

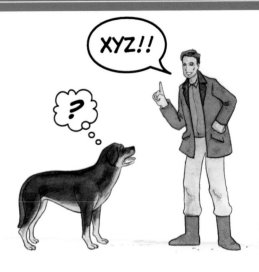

tempts to describe the way to you, the other person gradually starts to get impatient and finally irritated and angry. How would you feel?

A dog finds himself in just such a situation when we address him. He has to work out what you want from him, based on body language, gestures, facial expressions and possibly also mood transmission and previous experience. Not an easy task to achieve, which becomes almost impossible when he is also stressed due to your impatience, harshness or even punishment for apparently not following the command.

A dog that does not know what his owner wants from him reacts with stress to this expectations anxiety.

The owner can put the dog into an almost unbearable state of insecurity about what is expected from him when the owner behaves (from the dog's point of view) unpredictably. For example, sometimes the dog is allowed onto the sofa, other times he is "told off" for this. When he's at home with his owners, his begging is rewarded with food. But when visitors come he is scolded and told to go away. And so on and so on. The longer this situation of expectations anxiety lasts, the higher the stress levels are.

Failure
The dog is unsuccessful, fails at a task and is constantly frustrated in his efforts. He may also feel dissatisfaction coming from his owner.

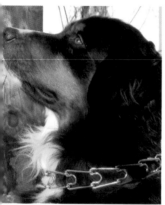

Harsh training methods

These can frighten and/or hurt the dog. Training a dog with sharp jerks on the leash causes injury to the vertebrae in his neck. The same is true for the use of spiked or choke collars, shock collars etc. Even leading the dog with an (on-the-surface) harmless-seeming head halter can, in the wrong hands, cause terrible physical and psychological damage. Yet, fear caused by harshly spoken commands and stiff body posture also belong on this list.

Spiked collars have no place in training!

Agility, dog dancing, obedience training

These types of dog sports have a very positive reputation and are associated with happy, co-operative dogs. However, the high pace and high performance pressure involved are causes for concern, particularly when the dog is expected to win a trophy for his owner.

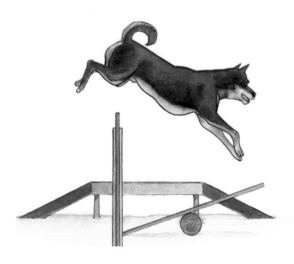

Even dog sports with positive reputations such as agility often cause stress as a result of the high pace and pressure to perform.

Schutzhund/ Protection Work

The physical strain and psychological pressure that builds up here stresses the dog. It is no surprise that many dogs working as service dogs have considerable problems with the kidneys, the cardiovascular, and digestive systems.

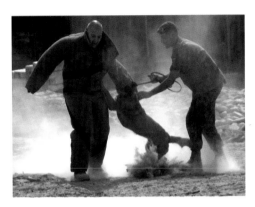

Puppy play groups

Even very worthwhile puppy play groups can turn into virtual "stress parties" if they are not professionally carried out and the dog is overwhelmed by the length of the play sessions, the size of the groups and the tasks he is expected to carry out.

The physical strain and psychological pressure of working dog training leads so often to stress in the dog that changed behavior and illness follow.

Worse still is that the puppy isn't just stressed temporarily, but badly organized play groups can have a serious impact on the dog's later behavior. We are often told about puppies being tired out but still being confronted with more and more stimuli. In some cases we've heard of puppies being awakened so that the play group could continue. This overburdening achieves exactly the opposite of what it sets out to do. The puppies start whining, some become quite irritated and aggressive and associate the experiences they have negatively because they are totally incapable of dealing with them. As a result, the same stimuli are interpreted as threatening, and the dog responds with either fearful and/or aggressive behavior.

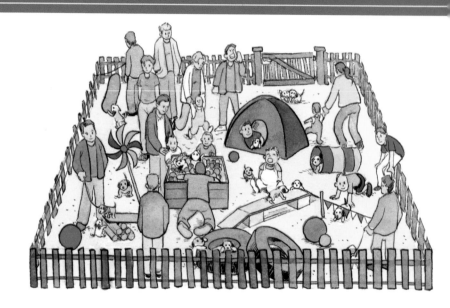

Even puppy play groups can turn into virtual "stress parties" if they are not professionally carried out and the dog is overwhelmed by the length of the play sessions, the size of the groups and the tasks he is expected to carry out.

Such startling overburdening and the resulting aggression often leads to bullying. This widely discussed topic should by no means be underestimated, as puppies that bully others "improve" this behavior every time they do so. On the other hand, the moment the victims of this bullying reach physical and mental maturity and are capable of defending themselves, they do the same – and with the same amount of vehemence as they were harassed before. In other words: bullying makes new bullies!

It is also noteworthy that these dogs later play very roughly and are often not very gentle with their play partners.

Never let your puppy be treated too roughly by other dogs. Help him if he needs your protection and wants to get away. Intervene in situations where he is being put upon by helping him out of the situation. Never listen to a trainer who tries to make you believe it's perfectly normal and that dogs sort it out among themselves!

Play is too rough and wild

Dogs get terribly stressed when play between two dogs or with a human gets too rough. This is often observed in puppies, which try to get away from the apparently playful situation by withdrawing, maybe by crawling under a bush or sofa. Adult dogs are also overwhelmed when the game is too frenetic and almost loaded with aggression.

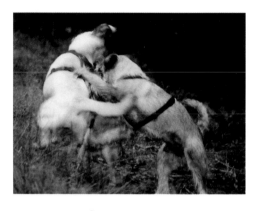

Men in particular may tend towards very rough and ready play because they believe this will toughen the dog up and that he must learn to stand up for himself. It is equally a widespread fallacy that puppies, young dogs or male dogs need this rough play in order to get a really good "work-out." Beware: this type of rough play forces the dog to defend himself in order to be finally left in peace. Mostly, at first, you see hectic defensive snapping in the air accompanied by growling. If the dog is still not left alone, the strain causes the dog to increase its defensive behavior. If he snaps at the owner, then the owner breaks off the game shouting at or scolding the dog, believing his punishment has taught the dog a lesson. And that is exactly what happens, the dog learns something – but something that he shouldn't learn: namely, that he will only be left alone if he defends himself physically.

Games that are too rough and too wild can stress the dog.

Similar situations occur also among dogs, so for this reason a heated game should be broken off.

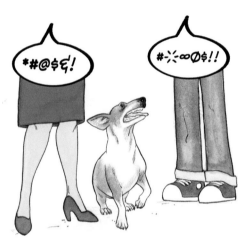

Violence, anger, irritation, and aggression around the dog
Arguments within his family, constant stress and angry voices in work areas, and people fighting all increase stress. The dog may not personally be the target of these outbursts, but he is stressed by the angry atmosphere.

Arguments and an angry atmosphere in the family stress the dog, even when he is not the target of the outburst.

Children
Up to a certain age, children are not capable of seeing dogs as independent beings with their own feelings, and so it can happen that they hold him tight, tug on him and treat him like some sort of replacement stuffed toy. Therefore, parents need to give their children suitable guidance. Even so, the dog may also get stressed by noises around him - wild and loud playing, noisy toys such as fire engines and trumpets, loud protests and crying.

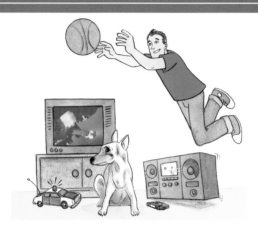

Too much coming and going at home

An "open door" with lots of new people coming and going, speaking to the dog, or simply just constant noise, can stress dogs as much as humans. We all need peace some time or another.

Too much emotional excitement

Whether positive or negative, emotional excitement stresses the dog. This can also include having to deal with unknown situations, even when they are not dangerous - exploring new things and processing stimuli can be exhausting. After all of this, the dog needs a sufficiently long period of quiet in order to work off the state of excitement.

A hectic household with many visitors, constant noise and playing children contains many stress factors.

Hunting games and races

In every game that involves chasing after a "prey" (such as a ball or a stick), the final sequence of hunting is playfully imitated.

In wild canines, the hunting of prey consists of a series of sequences. It begins with detecting the prey, something that often takes hours or even days. When the prey's scent is found or if the animal is seen, the scent is tracked and/or the animal is followed. Then it is stalked, possibly driven on so that it cannot rest, in order to bring it to the point of exhaustion. This process can also be drawn out over hours or even days. Finally, the attack follows. In order to have the necessary speed, aggression and power at its disposal, the body releases adrenalin. As described in our chapter on physiology, adrenalin optimises energy levels, the senses are sharpened, reactions are faster and the dog is more prepared to act aggressively.

It must be clearly pointed out that stick or ball games provoke this adrenalin release many times over and over, as the last of the above-mentioned prey sequences is constantly repeated. That is also one of the reasons why dogs get incredibly worked up during this type of game and are more ready to defend their "prey."

Additionally, in excessive races, where one dog tries to catch the other, the same mechanism is set in motion. If such a game lasts too long, it can lead to bullying or even turn into open aggression. Yet, even without this aggressive behavior, the dog is stressed by the physical changes associated with the release of adrenalin.

Un-doglike behavior (i.e., the dog can't understand)
For instance, the owner punishes the dog for apparently dominant behavior but the dog had behaved appropriately, given the circumstances. Due to a lack of knowledge, the owner had wrongly interpreted the situation.

EXAMPLE: *Ben, Mr M's two-year old Doberman male, was punished by his owner because he approached a German Shepherd, Sam, in a very stiffened, threatening way. Mr M. believed his dog was dominant and had to be brought down a peg or two. What Mr M. didn't know was that the very same German Shepherd, Sam, had attacked Ben only two days ago when out for a walk with Mrs M. So, Ben now had double the stress. He wasn't just confronted with his enemy, against whom he had to defend himself, but he was additionally punished by his owner, who had misunderstood the situation.*

A FURTHER EXAMPLE: *Bella, Mrs. B's rather withdrawn and anxious female Terrier cross, growled at all other females when they came too near. Mrs B.'s dog school told her that her dog was clearly dominant-aggressive against other dogs of the same gender (which was allegedly typical of Terriers) and should not be tolerated. Bella was also dominant towards Mrs B. when she did not immediately stop the behavior on command. For this reason, Mrs B would throw the dog onto its back into the sub-mission position. In reality, Bella was just anxious-aggressive as a result of previous bad experiences, as she was twice bitten by females so badly when she was a young dog that she had to be stitched. The two incidents occurred within five weeks of each other and, from then on, Bella attempted to keep other female dogs away from her through aggressive behavior. One cannot imagine the stress she was put under, both by the frightening situation and also from being punished by the most important person in her life.*

Discomfort

Stress can also be caused by physical discomfort, such as hunger, thirst, cold, warmth, noise, the lack of possibilities to relieve themselves, etc.

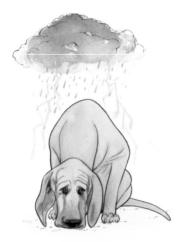

Bad weather

Thunder and lightening, storms, heavy rain, hail and natural catastrophes such as earthquakes. are common stressors for dogs.

Boarding kennels

The unusual surroundings, the strange smells and, above all, separation from the owner and the familiar home can trigger a stress reaction. Many dogs react with diarrhea or loss of appetite, going as far as refusing all food. Some become totally apathetic.

Many dogs are afraid of and stressed by bad weather and natural catastrophes.

At the vet's

Apart from the fact that the dog often has a physical complaint that makes the visit to the vet necessary, there are also other factors involved: the smell of the fear of the other animals present, unpleasant previous experiences of visiting the vet, the owner's anxiety, intruding the dog's individual space during examination, possibly painful treatment, to name but a few. Even when the vet makes every effort to be as gentle as possible with his patient, every dog is relieved when he can leave the clinic.

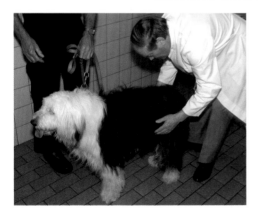

Unpleasant previous experiences, strange smells and a stranger intruding his individual space are just some of the stress factors involved in a visit to the vet.

The grooming salon

Stress is also triggered here by the many different noises (such as the clippers, the hair dryer) and intruding on the dog's individual space. Very few dogs enjoy being bathed and shampooed, standing on a table, hanging on the "gallows" and having their claws clipped. On top of this, the dog is often left alone by its owner during the appointment.

Fortunately, there are a growing number of grooming salons that visit their customers at home, take time with their four-legged clients and allow the owner to be present during the grooming session.

Exhibitions / fairs

There is no need to further explain why these events, taking place in huge halls with up to 5,000 visitors daily, are extremely exhausting and stressful for dogs - over-stimulation combined with a lack of mobility, hour-long car journey to and from the event.

Car journeys

Many dogs are totally overwhelmed by the images shooting past them at high speed, and bark constantly. Other dogs connect car trips with negative experiences such as visits to the vet or the separation from their mother and siblings and the previously familiar surroundings of the breeder's home, and so are afraid. Others become unwell and constantly dribble or vomit. All are stressed.

Reduced possibility of movement

Dogs are frequently stressed by being kept only on a chain or in a kennel, but also being kept only in the garden or always on the leash during walks, etc.

Loneliness/ boredom

Dogs also suffer from loneliness and boredom when they are too often left alone, are excluded from the family or have simply nothing to do.

Separation anxiety

This can surface in strange surroundings such as being chained outside a shop and left alone, or at home when the dog has not been trained to be alone. Adult dogs as well as puppies need to learn that they don't need to be afraid of such situations, and to trust that their owner will come back. If the dog hasn't yet been through this learning process, he can become afraid when the person he is close to is not there. It must be understood that for this social animal it is not normal to be separated from the social group and left alone.

High population concentration

When too many dogs are kept too close to each other and don't have enough opportunity to withdraw, and their individual space is not respected, this will result in stress. This is true when there are too many dogs in the house, in animal shelters, research labs or similar. Often, stress-induced bullying and increasingly aggressive behavior occurs. How long a dog can tolerate and/or compensate for this situation depends on many factors: How confined is the situation? Is there potential for conflict within the group? Does the group stay constant or does it constantly change due to some dogs being found homes, or given away? How old is the dog? How healthy is he? What breed is he?

Bad canine mix in one house
This does not necessarily mean that there are serious fights between the dogs. Even constantly having to get out of each other's way or creeping around each other causes enormous stress, just as it does in humans. Imagine you have to share the place where you live, your home, the place you can withdraw to, with someone you don't actually like and with whom there is constantly an undertone of conflict. Not a nice thought. Yet, many owners place their dog in just such a situation. Another dog is brought into the household without any thought for the likes and dislikes of the other dog. Often the dog responds with stress symptoms such as diarrhea, vomiting, restlessness or also apathy.

The dog is suffocated by the owner's emotional needs
Some dogs are not just totally treated as little humans and not seen as dogs, but also showered with love and attention, only to be then completely ignored because the owner is busy – this hot/cold emotional shower leaves no dog untouched.

In exactly the same way, too frequent or too little physical contact triggers stress
Small dogs such as the Cavalier King Charles Spaniel, the Chihuahua as well as puppies are constantly lifted up, stroked and kissed. If you watch the dog's expressions, body language and the calming signals he displays, you will quickly see that it is all too much for him. Other dogs on the other hand receive far too little physical contact and are hardly ever stroked. If a dog is constantly frustrated in his search for attention, this also triggers stress.

Too many or almost no rules in daily life.
Both can overwhelm the dog. A dog that is constantly ordered around and told what he can and cannot do gets stressed very quickly. At the same time, a dog that has no rules and where the security or routine in daily interaction with us is missing, does not feel at all happy.

Bad dog-human suitability
The dog cannot fulfill his human's requirements because the dog's basic needs do not fit into the circumstances in which he is living An example is a Weimaraner or German Long Hair that was bred to be a hunting dog but is kept in a three-room apartment and is only walked twice daily around the block by an owner who works full-time. Another example is a Basset with breeding-induced crippled legs that is taken by its owner for long walks through the mountains. This list could go on. The only thing to consider here is how it would be possible to convince people to not choose their future partner according to how cute they look.

Notes

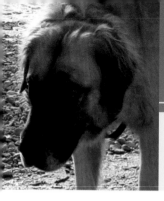

SURVEY ON THE LIVING CONDITIONS OF DOGS AND ON STRESS SYMPTOMS

INTRODUCTION TO THE SURVEY

The questionnaire

The survey contains 40 questions on the daily life of dogs and on possible stress symptoms. It was distributed among friends with dogs and clients as well as being made publicly available on the internet. 224 surveys were filled out, returned, and evaluated. The returned forms showed that some of the participants had more than the average involvement with dogs as they were praticing dog trainers or veterinary advisers.

The 40 questions are divided into various sections. The first part covers general questions about the dog, such as breed, age and gender.

In the second part there are questions about the dog's living conditions. Where is the dog during the day? How often and for how long does he/she go for walks? How frequently does he/she have the opportunity to run free, meet other dogs and how many hours a day does he/she sleep?

In the third part there are a few questions about any current illnesses.

The fourth and final part contains a list of symptoms and behaviors that could be indicators of stress.

Method for the allocation of stress points

The survey contains fifteen possible stress indicators. The participants were asked to enter how frequently each behavior occurred. They could decide between:

☐ never   ☐ seldom
☐ frequently, or ☐ often

For the purposes of statistical evaluation, each answer was awarded the following points:

For the first two points (restlessness, hyperactivity)
    never = 0 points; seldom= 5 points
    frequently = 10 points ; often= 20 points.

For all other questions
    never = 0 points; Seldom = 1 point
    frequently = 5 points ; often = 10 points.

Finally, the total stress points for each dog were calculated.

Evaluation of the stress points

By way of reference for all of the evaluations, an average value for the 224 dogs was established. All stress points were added together and divided by the total number of dogs. As a result, the average total of stress points for all the dogs was established as 22.85. Where a clearly higher or lower value for a particular group is observed, it can be assumed that the stress burden is clearly higher or lower than the average.

RESULTS OF THE SURVEY

BREED

The first question was about breed. The answers were divided into groups. The average stress points for the individual breeds were compared with each other.

	Breed	Number (per cent)	Average stress points
1	Cross breed / mongrel	71 (31.7%)	22.4
2	Working dogs*	36 (16.1%)	30.2
3	Herding dogs (mostly the Border Collie)	35 (15.6%)	24.4
4	Livestock guardian dogs	18 (8.0%)	13.9
5	Poodle and other lap dogs	17 (7.6%)	21.4
6	Terriers	14 (6.2%)	15.9
7	Retrievers	13 (5.8%)	20.8
8	Hunting dogs	12 (5.4%)	23.1
9	Sighthounds	4 (1.8%)	15.3
10	Nordic dogs	4 (1.8%)	29.5

As defined here, Workings dogs refers to those breeds which are traditionally involved in Schutzhund (protection /tracking dog) sports such as the German Shepherd, Giant Schnauzer, Boxer, Dobermann, Rottweiler, Hovawart, Airedale Terrier, Bouvier and Malinois.

The evaluation in chart form:

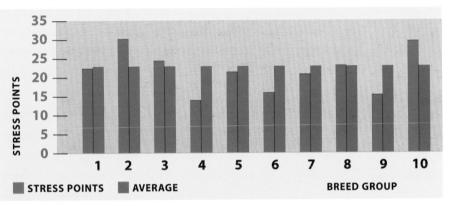

Our evaluation indicates that working dogs (see page 62) bear the greatest burden of stress. The cause cannot be found in dog sports alone; as the following evaluation shows, the practice of a type of dog sport does not necessarily influence the stress levels to which the dog is exposed. More decisive is how - and how often - the dog is trained. One reason for the result above is more likely to be that these breeds have a lower stress threshold than others, resulting more easily in stress due to the dog's tendency to over-react. With this in mind, the comparison with livestock guardian dogs is very interesting, dogs known for their very high threshold. The average value for livestock guardian dogs was 13.9, lying clearly below the overall average of 22.85.

GENDER

The question on gender brought the following result:

	Number of dogs	Average stress points
Male dogs	107	24.55
Neutered male dogs	36	27.10
	(33.6% of male dogs)	
Female dogs	109	21.44
Spayed female dogs	59	23.88
	(54.1% of female dogs)	

Of the 224 dogs, 107 were male and 109 female. Eight of the participants did not answer this question.

Both neutered male dogs as well as spayed females showed a higher stress point average than the total number of male and female dogs.

A typically held explanation for this is that the altered social behavior of other non-castrated dogs towards castrated dogs raises stress. It is often reported that non-neutered male dogs do not treat neutered dogs as male dogs anymore but as aromatic females, leading to increased mounting.

The more plausible explanation is that castration is often used as a magic remedy for "solving" behavioral problems. In all probability this means that castrated dogs show raised stress levels even before castration, and that castration is obviously not really suited to solving the problem. It was further apparent that males show a higher average stress point value than females.

Summary of other survey results

- 137 dogs (61.2%) came to their families as puppies.
- 35 dogs (15.6%) were younger than 1 year old when they came to their owners.
- 49 dogs (21.9%) were already adults when they were rehomed
- 204 of the 224 dogs (91.1%) stay in the house during the day.
- 157 dogs (70.1%) are allowed to sleep in the bedroom during the night.
- 4 dogs (1.8%) are kept in a kennel.

RESTING PHASES

We asked how many hours a day the dogs sleep or rest.

The following table shows the result:

Number of hours the dog rests	Number of dogs	Average stress points
Up to 10 hours	23 (10.3%)	27.0
11 to 13 hours	28 (12.5%)	25.0
14 to 16 hours	78 (34.8%)	24.4
17 to 19 hours	72 (21.6%)	21.6
20 hours or more	23 (10.3%)	14.7

The evaluation in chart form:

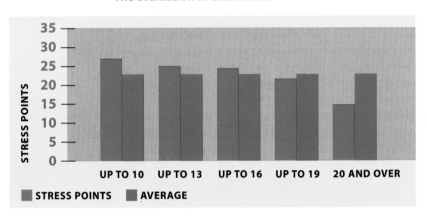

Dogs that sleep or rest fewer than 17 hours per day have a much higher stress point value than the overall average. We must therefore draw from this that every dog should have the opportunity to sleep or rest 17 hours daily.

As the stress point total rises with every hour less of sleep, lack of rest can be seen as a stress symptom. In other words, if the dog owner encourages excessive activity, this can trigger stress problems in the dog. For this reason, every dog owner should make sure that days of heightened activity should be followed by a generous resting phase.

BEING ALONE

The next point in the evaluation looks at the question of whether and how long the dog has to stay alone. Does the dog regularly have to stay at home on its own? If so, how many hours on average?

Dog must regularly stay alone for	Number of dogs	Stress points average
0 hours	76 (34.4%)	22.1
1 hour	30 (13.4%)	23.2
2 to 3 hours	37 (16.5%)	22.6
4 to 5 hours	46 (20.8%)	21.4
6 hours or over	35 (15.6%)	26.3

The evaluation in chart form:

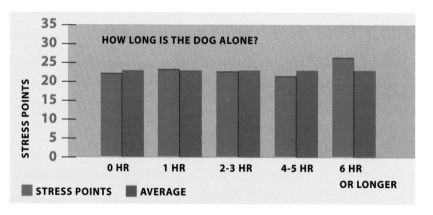

If the dog is left alone for no more than 5 hours daily the established stress point value lies within the 22.85 overall average for all participating dogs. The lowest value of 21.4 is found among the group that has to stay alone for 4 to 5

hours daily. A possible explanation could be that these dogs have enough time to sleep and rest, something that turned out to be of great importance. A pre-condition for this is of course that the dog has learned how to stay alone step by step and that he does not feel panic or fear the moment his human leaves the house.

At 26.3, the value for the group that has to stay alone for 6 hours or more is much higher than the average, leading to the conclusion that this time span is too long.

WALKING THE DOG

The next question concerned walk routines.

The first question established how long in total the dog was walked. The following table shows the result:

Hours	Number of dogs	Stress points average
Up to 2 hours	116 (51.8%)	21.8
3 hours	82 (36.6%)	23.1
More than 3 hours	26 (11.6%)	26.9

At 23.1, the established stress point value for those dogs walked for 3 hours is only slightly higher than the average value for all dogs. The 26.9 value for the group of dogs walked for longer than 3 hours is much higher than the comparative value. So it is easy to suspect that long walks and being taken everywhere puts strain on many dogs. The evaluation indicates therefore the necessity for a balance between sufficient sleep/resting phases and joint activities. A deficit in the sleep and resting phases leads just as easily to stress as does too much activity.

The evaluation in chart form:

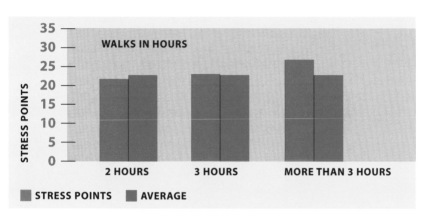

RUNNING FREE AND CONTACT WITH OTHER DOGS

The next questions involved the opportunity for the dog to run free and contact with other dogs.

Is your dog allowed to run free?	Does he/ she come into contact with other dogs?	Number of dogs	Stress points average
yes	yes	126	21.4
yes	no	43	26.3
no	yes	20	23.6
no	no	35	23.4

This table shows that dogs that regularly meet dogs while running free demonstrate the lowest stress points - a hardly surprising result.

The second row represents dogs that have the opportunity to run free but have no regular contact with other dogs. At 26.3, the stress point value here is much higher than in the first group.

Rows 3 and 4 deal with dogs that are mostly led on the leash. They show a higher stress point value than dogs that are mostly allowed to run free and have contact with other dogs.

In summary, it must be clearly stated that being allowed to run free and meet other dogs is obviously essential for this run-loving social animal.

THREATS
The next question examined situations the dog feels threatening, leading to fearful or aggressive behavior.

The following table shows the result:

The dog feels threatened	Number of dogs	Stress points average
Never or seldom	157 (70.1%)	18.5
Frequently or often	67 (29.%)	33.1

The evaluation in chart form:

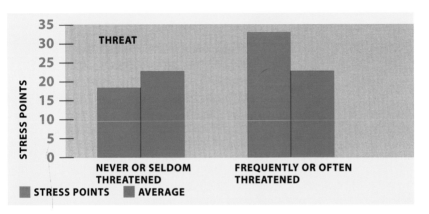

The average value for dogs that feel frequently or often threatened is 33.1 This is an almost 50% increase on the reference value. This shows that the feeling of being threatened – being afraid and possibly reacting aggressively to a threat – represents a serious problem for these dogs and considerably raises stress levels.

GAMES AND DOG SPORTS

The first question of this section was whether the dog owner regularly plays with his dog. The second question asks whether children under twelve regularly play with the dog. The table shows the result:

Regularly plays with dog	Number of dogs	Stress points average
Yes	193 (86.1%)	23.7
No	31 (13.9%)	17.8
Children also play with dog	38 (17.0%)	23.8

The average stress point value for dogs that are played with lies only slightly above the reference value. The surprising aspect was that the result shows it is apparently not decisive whether children are involved or not. It must however be taken into consideration that most of the survey participants are experienced dog owners who (presumably) observe and guide their children during play. The authors would like to point out that the observation and guidance of children during play with dogs is absolutely essential. By way of example, please read Mona's case history (page 114).

When the values for the dogs that are played with are compared with the group whose owners do not regularly play with their dogs, you will notice that their value of 17.8 is much lower. This makes it clear that regular play can raise the dog's stress levels. Naturally, it also depends how often, how long and what types of games are played.

The next question looks at the issue of whether the dog trains in or takes part in dog sports, and what form these take. The following table shows the result:

Number of different dog sports	Number of dogs	Stress points average
None	115 (51.3%)	22.5
1 or 2	85 (37.9%)	22.4
3 or more	23 (10.3%)	24.9

The results show that whether the dog takes part in a dog sport or not has obviously no bearing on the stress burden. The question of whether he takes part in different forms of dog sport also seems to be of little relevance. The stress point value only rises when the number of activities engaged in reaches 3 or 4. By such extensive and intensive training it seems to be difficult not to overburden the dog. As so often is the case, it is a question of how often, with which methods and - not least - how ambitiously the dog is trained. It is recommended that you look out for stress symptoms. If necessary, reduce training times and place fewer demands on your dog.

ILLNESSES

In the next 3 questions, we aimed to specify the illnesses, with questions about allergies, skin diseases and digestive problems and/or diarrhea.

The following table shows the result:

	Number of dogs	Stress points average
Never or seldom ill	200 (89.3%)	21.9
Frequently or often ill	24 (10.7%)	30.8
Dog suffers from allergies	30 (13.4%)	23.7
Dog has skin problems	18 (8.0%)	26.3
Dog has digestive problems/ diarrhea	26 (11.6%)	35.5

The evaluation in chart form:

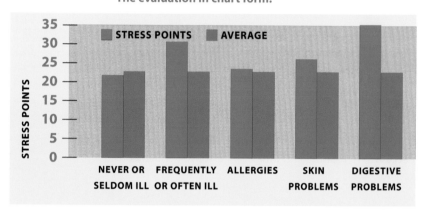

It is nice to discover that almost 90% of the dog owners stated that their dog had no health problems.

The average stress point value of the dogs that were frequently or often ill is 30.8 and therefore relatively high in comparison with the reference value for all dogs (22.85). This is of course no wonder, as every illness that affects the organism causes stress.

The group of dogs suffering from digestive problems or diarrhea has a particularly high stress point value. At 35.5 it is the highest of all the established statistical values. It can be concluded from this that digestive problems and diarrhea are closely connected to stress and should also be seen as a stress symptom. Indeed, stories abound in veterinary clinics and dog schools of dogs reacting with digestive problems to stressful situations.

This group of dogs was analyzed in more detail in order to more closely examine the connection between stress and digestive problems. Of the 26 dogs with more frequent digestive problems, 18 (69.2%) indicated a higher than average stress point value. This means that more than two thirds of these dogs are exposed to a higher than average stress burden. For this reason, we examined to what extent the previously established stress releasing factors applied to the 18 dogs. In the following table, each individual dog is characterized by whether he/she has less than 17 hours rest, is alone longer than 5 hours per day, goes for walks for 3 hours or more, or frequently feels threatened.

It became apparent that at least one of the stress triggering factors applies to each of these dogs. 77.8% of the dogs sleep or rest less than 17 hours, 38.9% have to stay alone for 5 hours per day and 61.1% go for walks 3 hours or longer per day. The owners of 10 dogs (55.6%) stated that their dog felt frequently or often threatened. This information shows clearly that stress must be considered a triggering factor in dogs that frequently suffer from digestive problems, especially when no physical cause can be found through veterinary examination. It is recommended that the living conditions of these dogs be examined and that you become aware of any possible stress releasing factors.

	Less than 17 hours sleep	More than 5 hours alone daily	3 or more hours walks	Dog feels frequently or often threatened
1	no	no	YES	no
2	YES	no	YES	YES
3	no	YES	no	no
4	YES	YES	YES	no
5	YES	no	no	YES
6	YES	YES	YES	no
7	YES	YES	YES	YES
8	YES	no	no	no
9	YES	no	YES	no
10	YES	no	YES	YES
11	no	no	YES	no
12	YES	no	no	no
13	YES	no	no	YES
14	no	YES	no	YES
15	YES	no	no	YES
16	YES	no	YES	YES
17	YES	YES	YES	YES
18	YES	YES	YES	YES
	77.8%	**38.9%**	**61.1%**	**55.6%**

STATISTICS OF THE INDIVIDUAL STRESS SYMPTOMS

The last part of the survey contains a list of 15 possible stress symptoms. The participants were asked to mark each possible symptom and note how often they had observed this in their dog.

The table shows the number of dogs where the answers "frequently" or "often" were marked:

Stress symptom	Number	As a percentage
Restlessness	31	13.8%
Hyperactivity	35	15.6%
Very frequent display of calming signals	87	38.8%
Aggressive or anxious behavior	49	21.9%
Compulsive behavior	17	7.6%
Displacement activity	36	16.1%
Lack of concentration	42	18.8%
Dog appears "distant"	24	10.7%
Muscular problems	12	5.4%
Panting	25	11.1%
Underweight	13	5.8%
Excessive self-grooming	17	7.6%
Destructiveness	11	4.9%
Frequent barking or whining	64	28.6%
Very frequent urinating	35	15.6%

Final observations

It would be interesting to set the results of this survey off against a larger number of participants and to also ask much more detailed questions. The 224 participants cannot guarantee a completely thorough examination of all aspects of the subject. For example, only 4 Nordic breed owners took part. Although during the evaluation these 4 dogs matched in many areas, such a small number does not allow for any generalised statements about the Nordic breeds.

Nevertheless, we found the results very revealing. Some we expected – e.g., the important influence on the dog's psychological and physical balance of sleep and rest phases, the opportunity to run free, and for social contact. We were also previously aware of the direct connection between stress and various illnesses.

We were however surprised by other results - for instance, that so many of those questioned believed their dogs to be healthy. We presume that this statement was affected by the owner's subjective feelings towards their dog. That means that some of them did not see the dog's illness as such anymore, as they had already got used to the dog's symptoms. Many owners found it "normal" for their dog to frequently have diarrhea - nevertheless, this is still an illness.

We were also surprised that many dogs can obviously stay for up to 5 hours on their own without problems. Separation anxiety and the associated destruction of interior fittings or hour-long barking are one of the main reasons for dogs being given away.

On the following pages you will find the questions used for this survey. It was created by Martina Scholz for an educational event, sent off and evaluated. Particular thanks go out to those who took the time to fill it out and send it back for evaluation.

SURVEY QUESTIONS

1. **Questions about the dog, daily routine and holding conditions**

1.1. Dog
Breed:
Male or female:

Is the dog spayed/neutrered?
☐ yes   ☐ no

How old is the dog?
At what age did he/she come to you?

1.2. An average day
Where is the dog mainly kept during the day?
☐ in the garden   ☐ in the house
☐ in a kennel

Where does the dog sleep at night?
☐ in a kennel   ☐ in a hallway
☐ in the living room   ☐ in yours or the children's
                            bedroom
How many hours does the dog sleep or doze in total
(day and night)?

How many hours is the dog normally alone?

How many hours maximum is the dog alone?

Does your dog follow you around?
☐ yes   ☐ no

Or does he/she doze in a favorite place
during the day?

☐ yes ☐ no

How long do you go for walks with your dog?

☐ up to one hour ☐ up to two hours
☐ up to three hours ☐ more than three hours

How often do you go for walks every day?

☐ once ☐ two to three times
☐ more than three times

During these walks, the dog

☐ is mostly on the leash ☐ mostly runs free

During these walks, the dog has

☐ frequent contact with other dogs
☐ seldom contact with other dogs

Does your dog ever feel threatened?
Does he/ she show aggression or react anxiously?

☐ never ☐ seldom
☐ frequently ☐ often

1.3. Activities with the dog

Do you regularly play with your dog?
☐ yes   ☐ no

Do children (up to 12 years of age) play with the dog?
☐ yes   ☐ no

Do you take part in a dog sport?
☐ yes   ☐ no
If so, which?

How many hours a day is your dog active?

1.4. Your dog's health

How frequently is your dog ill?
☐ never   ☐ seldom
☐ frequently   ☐ often

Does your dog suffer from allergies?
☐ yes   ☐ no

Does your dog have skin ailments?
☐ yes   ☐ no

Does your dog have frequent diarrhea or often vomit?
☐ yes   ☐ no

2. Have you ever observed the following behavior in your dog?

Restlessness, the dog cannot settle down
☐ never   ☐ seldom
☐ frequently   ☐ often

The dog is never tired, plays till he/ she "collapses"
☐ never   ☐ seldom
☐ frequently   ☐ often

Very frequent display of calming signals
(yawning, blinking, looking away, etc)
☐ never   ☐ seldom
☐ frequently   ☐ often

Inappropriately aggressive or nervous behavior
☐ never   ☐ seldom
☐ frequently   ☐ often

Compulsive behavior
(e.g. adult dog chasing his/her own tail)
☐ never   ☐ seldom
☐ frequently   ☐ often

Displacement activity, e.g. biting the leash
☐ never   ☐ seldom
☐ frequently   ☐ often

Poor concentration
☐ never   ☐ seldom
☐ frequently   ☐ often

Dog appears "distant"
- [ ] never
- [ ] frequently
- [ ] seldom
- [ ] often

Trembling, tense muscles
- [ ] never
- [ ] frequently
- [ ] seldom
- [ ] often

Panting, although not exhausted or warm
- [ ] never
- [ ] frequently
- [ ] seldom
- [ ] often

Underweight
- [ ] yes
- [ ] no

Excessive self-grooming
- [ ] never
- [ ] frequently
- [ ] seldom
- [ ] often

Destructiveness
- [ ] never
- [ ] frequently
- [ ] seldom
- [ ] often

Barking, whining, etc
- [ ] never
- [ ] frequently
- [ ] seldom
- [ ] often

Very frequent urination
- [ ] never
- [ ] frequently
- [ ] seldom
- [ ] often

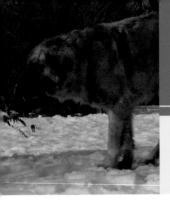

THE ANTI-STRESS PROGRAM (ASP)

By way of introduction to this chapter it must be stated that there is no magic remedy for stressed dogs! As mentioned on a number of occasions there are considerable individual differences between how much and what type of stress a dog can cope with before his/her health suffers or behavioral changes are observed. This depends on socialization, on his/ her state of health, age, previous experiences, surroundings and many other factors.

The surroundings are of particular importance as no canine living in the wild is exposed to as many stress-triggering situations as the domestic dog. Even though, in the course of domestication, resistance to stress improved markedly, it is still the case that dogs have never before lived in such surroundings where they have to tolerate so many (in many cases constantly repeated) stressful situations.

In this respect, it is often difficult to work out which of the known factors is the one that the dog is exposed to. Typically a series of individual factors cause an over-spill, so to speak. It is therefore important to not just examine individual events but also to get the full picture of the dog's complete surroundings, daily routine, fundamental relationship to the owner or to other human or animal members of the household. To do this, we use the following questionnaire:

> **SORRY, BUT THERE IS NO MAGIC REMEDY FOR STRESSED DOGS!**

QUESTIONNAIRE

Your personal details, which will not be passed on to third parties

Name:

Address:

Tel / Mobile:

Email:

Questions about your dog:

Name: Gender:

Breed: Age:

neutered/spayed: ☐ yes   ☐ no

If your dog is neutered/spayed, please answer the following questions:

When was your dog neutered/spayed?

How old was your dog when this occurred?

Why was your dog neutered/spayed?

For females: did your dog previously give birth?

If so, please enter how often, at what age and how many puppies per litter?

If your female dog is not spayed, when was she last in season?

_____

Questions about your dog's health condition:

Is your dog vaccinated?   yes ☐   no ☐
_____
(Date and type of vaccination)

Is your dog wormed?   ☐ yes, on   ☐ no

Does your dog suffer from a chronic illness?   ☐ yes ☐ no

If so, which? _____

Is he/she regularly given medicine   ☐ yes ☐ no

If so, which? _____
                        (please enter the dose)

When was he/ she first given the medicine? _____

How does your dog behave in a veterinary clinic?

_____

_____

_____

_____

_____

General questions about your dog:

Where did you get your dog? _____

How long has he/she lived with you? _____

How old was he/she when he/she came to you? _____

Did he/she have previous owners? ☐ yes, _____ owner(s) ☐ no

What do you know about your dog's previous history? _____

_____

_____

_____

How many people live with you?

_____ Adults, _____ children, aged _____

Are there other dogs in your household? ☐ yes ☐ no

If so, how many? _____
(age, breed, gender)

Are there other animals in your household? ☐ yes ☐ no

If so, which and how many? _____

_____

Is this your first dog?　　　　　　☐ yes　　☐ no

Why did you choose this breed?

_____

_____

Why did you decide on this particular gender?

_____

_____

For what reasons did you decide to get a dog?

_____

_____

_____

Did all of the family members agree with the decision to get a dog?

_____

Where is the dog when you travel without him/her?

_____

Where/ how do you live?

_____

(city / village / apartment / house / garden)

Questions on the dog's training:

Have you ever attended a dog school? ☐ yes ☐ no

If so, which commands did your dog learn there? _____

_____

_____

_____

Did your dog enjoy going there? yes ☐ no ☐

Did you enjoy going there? ☐ yes ☐ no

How often did you go for training? _____

_____

Please put a check for any of the following types of training you have already done with your dog:

☐ Obedience
☐ Companion dog training
☐ Protection work
☐ Degility
☐ Subordination training
☐ Training with horses
☐ Clicker training
☐ Training with a head halter
☐ Other aversive training methods
☐ Shock collar training

☐ Dog dancing
☐ Stamina training
☐ Agility
☐ Tellington Touch / ground work
☐ Guard dog training
☐ Rescue dog training
☐ Throw chain / disc training
☐ Coyote call training*
☐ others

*Where the handler uses a coyote pipe to attract coyotes.

Questions on the dog's typical day:

Where is the dog usually kept?

_____

_____

Where is his/ her favorite resting place / where does he/ she sleep?

_____

_____

Who goes with him/her for walks?

_____

_____

How long and how often?
☐ on the leash   ☐ he/ she runs free
☐ run free, or on the leash depending on the situation

Does your dog pull on the leash?   yes ☐   no ☐

Do you play with your dog? How long, how often, and how?

_____

_____

_____

Does your dog stay alone at
home without problems?   ☐ yes   ☐ no

If not, what does he/ she do?

_____

_____

_____

How often and for how long must your dog stay at home alone?

_____

Are there situations when your dog appears to be stressed?

_____

_____

_____

Questions about your dog's food:

How often do you feed your dog daily?

What is your dog's main meal of the day?

_____

Where do you feed your dog?

_____

(kitchen, garden, hallway, etc)

How does he/ she behave during feeding?

_____

_____

_____

Does your dog receive chews or treats?

☐ yes, _____   ☐ no
    (chews, milk drops, sausage, cheese, etc.)

Does your dog have any food allergies/intolerances?
_____

_____

_____

How long does your dog rest after feeding?
_____

_____

Questions about your dog's sleeping habits / resting periods:

How many hours a day does your dog normally sleep or slumber?
_____

_____

Does he/ she have vivid dreams?
_____

_____

Is your dog a light or deep sleeper?
_____

_____

Does your dog sleep in his/her favorite place or elsewhere?
_____

_____

Do you have problems living with your dog?

_____

_____

What does he/she do exactly?

_____

_____

_____

Was there a "key experience" or a particular trigger that
caused this behavior?

_____

_____

When did you first notice this behavior?

_____

What have you done about it so far?

_____

_____

How would you like the dog to behave differently to the way he does?

_____

What goal/s would you like to achieve through training with us? Is there anything that is particularly important for you? Or something that you and your dog would particularly enjoy?

_____

_____

_____

_____

_____

What do you like most about your dog?

_____

_____

_____

_____

_____

Thank you for your co-operation!

With the answers from the questionnaire and the information that we get from observing the dog and the owner, we can form a relatively complete picture of the dog's living circumstances and whether – and to what extent – the dog is stressed. To do this it is necessary to observe the dog while he/she goes for walks in both a familiar and also in an unknown area, how he/she behaves at home and in the car, etc. We try to find out which factors lead to which symptoms.

The next step is then to reduce as many of the stress triggering factors as possible. Here it is absolutely crucial to make sure that we do not attempt to change too many things at once in the dog's social environment because this itself could trigger stress. Many things must be changed step by step and dogs that are wound up through physical exertion – in the same way as top athletes – must be brought slowly back to normal activity levels. For this reason an anti-stress program does not just run over days but often over weeks and months before any noticeable improvements can be seen. Despite the changes in the living circumstances, the body needs time to react and for the stress hormone levels to normalize. In our experience, animals that have suffered from stress over a long (or very long) period generally also need a long period to work off this stress. It is important to speak about this with the dog owner right at the beginning so that he/she does not become frustrated when no major changes can be seen in the first few days.

The following case studies show what an anti-stress program can look like. The dogs and humans described are real. The owners of Diego, Mona, Wolfgang and Bernd came as clients to Clarissa von Reinhardts' dog school. In some cases we have changed the names at the request of the person concerned.

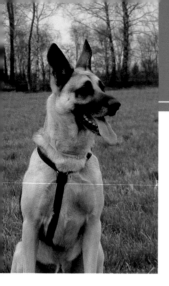

DIEGO

Diego is a large, slim German Shepherd cross who first came to my dog school in February 2002. His owner, Ms Trobisch, told me that she first saw Diego in an animal shelter in January 1998. According to the animal shelter workers, he was then about one year old. The only information about his earlier life was that the previous owner kept him tied with a short chain to the central heating in his apartment. The man had not looked after the large, lively dog at all well. Diego was underweight, nervous, very afraid of and insecure towards other dogs, but friendly towards humans.

Ms Trobisch decided to give the dog a home. At first, Diego suffered such terrible separation anxiety that his owner could not even go to the restroom without him. The moment he was left alone, he destroyed the apartment. He scratched the doors, ravaged the furniture, tore the blinds down. If he had to stay alone in the car, he destroyed the interior. Despite his great need for proximity, from the very beginning he shyed from touch and seemed very uncomfortable when his owner came too close. He let himself be stroked for a short time and then moved away.

A year after taking him out of the animal shelter, the opportunity arose for Ms Trobisch to work from home. She used this time to work intensively with Diego on his separation anxiety. For such training, it is essential that the feeling of being left alone is never allowed to surface. This means of course that, at the beginning, the dog cannot be left alone for one moment. The dog gets slowly accustomed to being alone, starting with a few seconds, then later minutes and finally longer periods of time. Diego's training was successful. One year later, when Ms Trobisch began to work away from home again, Diego could stay alone at home without any problems.

In 1999, private and professional reasons obliged Ms Trobisch to move home four times with Diego in tow, which of course put an enormous strain on him. Ms Trobisch went for long walks with him and played ball with him on a field up to four hours (!) a day. At first I could not really imagine this happening but she actually threw him a ball again and again because she believed he should have movement and fun. She had also been told that such a lively dog really needed a good work out…

Ms Trobisch decided on a second dog in September 2000 after being advised to do so by a trainer whose dog school she was attending. The trainer's argument was that such a lively dog as Diego needed an equally lively partner, and that both would mutually tire each other out. A well balanced, quiet dog would not be able to keep up with his temperament. so Ms Trobisch opted for a Dalmatian. Anna came as a 12-week old puppy to Ms Trobisch and her partner. She was quite anxious and withdrawn. It was touching to see that Diego looked after her but, he then started to attack other dogs that frightened Anna by coming too close to her.

The excessive ball-play also created problems – Diego succombed very quickly to prey aggression. On top of this, Ms Trobisch recognized that Diego was sometimes so worked up that he didn't even notice that other dogs had come near him. When they stood directly in front of him, he dropped

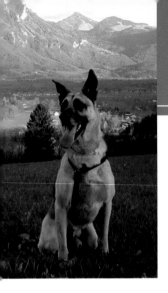

the ball and jumped on them. Due to his size and strength it didn't take long before he had pinned the other dog under him, although he had not yet bitten. Ms Trobisch didn't want to tolerate this behavior and turned once again to her dog school. She was advised to put little Anna in a young dog group because she was so insecure and needed to learn how to cope for herself. The dogs in this group were allowed to play together and certain commands were practiced. It was recommended that Diego undergo individual training with the goal of getting him so fixated on his beloved ball that he would no longer be interested in anything else. The argument was that he would then be much easier to control. Diego did ten hours of individual training in which he learned basic obedience commands such as "sit," "down," stay," "heel," and "here," and would be rewarded for correctly carrying out the commands by having his ball thrown to him. The command "stay" caused major problems at first because, when the ball was thrown to him and he was supposed to stay put, he went crazy. He barked, tried to break free, jumped up, and behaved crazily. Unless he was tied onto something, he was uncontrollable. Trainer and owner were, as a result, filled with pride when, after countless repeats, it finally worked. When Diego received the command to "stay," he stayed sitting. When he got the command to fetch, he shot off like a rocket in order to get the ball. Towards other dogs, however, he was increasingly more nervous and ready to attack.

It gradually became clear to Ms Trobisch that she and her trainer had obviously different goals for Diego's training. Ms Trobisch wanted her dog to be calmer and more sociable. The trainer's goal was control over the dog. After consultation, the decision was made for Diego to do a training course with six to seven other dogs in order to improve his social behavior. The size of the designated training ground was 250 square meters. Diego went crazy the moment he saw the other leashed dogs. Ms Trobisch had great difficulty holding him because he jumped up on her, barked constantly and she could not get through to him. As the training ground was so small and also had an agility course built on it, there was no possibility of taking him to one side in order to calm him down. Instead, he was kept on as short a leash as possible, which made him even more worked up. Ms Trobisch had the feeling that both she and her dog were overwhelmed by the situation. The trainer advised both of them to take a nerve remedy before each visit to the training ground!

However, the drama started well before, when they were on the way to the training ground. Diego knew full well which days and at which times his owner would take him for training. During the entire journey he barked and scratched on the windows and upholstery. When they were finally at the training ground, he didn't want to get out and tried to run away. Conversely, at the end of training he pulled like mad back to the car. The dog could hardly be held any more and so Ms Trobisch started to park in other places so that her dog would not notice where they were going. She walked a bit with him before she reached the training ground and made sure they were the first to arrive. Ms Trobisch felt this made the situation easier for him to bear.

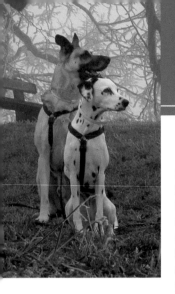

Because she still had great difficulty holding Diego, the trainer advised her to fit him with a head halter in order to have better control over him. Previously, he had been prone to over-reacting. He would shoot forward without warning and snap at any dog that came too close to him on the extremely small training ground. His owner described his eyes at such times as flickering and hectic and she felt she could not guarantee the safety of the other dogs. Indeed, the head halter worsened the situation. The moment it was put on Diego, he stood with a cowering posture, his tail clamped between his legs, displaying calming signals – a sorrowful sight. He tried on many occasions with his front paws to get the head halter off, for which he was scolded.

Weeks and months went by and Diego successfully got through three training courses, whereby the definition of the word "successful" is a moot point here. He had passed all tests, had even won a trophy and had mastered all of the commands to perfection. Yet, he was more nervous and more aggressive than ever before. Ms Trobisch told me that, as a result of the considerable strain she was under, she was often very unfair to her dog. When her patience and physical energy left her, she screamed at him, jerked hard on the leash, forced him down onto the floor and held his muzzle hard. She was unhappy about this and felt as if she was really being unfair to her dog.

Finally, she was advised to enter Diego in a new course - obedience and agility. As he was so energetic he needed to be kept busy and given enough movement. As mentioned earlier, the agility course was built on a 250 square meters area. The training took place with either Diego leashed, or all other dogs put on the leash and waiting on the edge of the course while the unleashed Diego ran and/or raced through the course. As he was too worked up to take any treats, he was rewarded once again with having his ball thrown to him.

In the meantime, Anna was one and a half years old. She had herself not only passed all group training courses but also three agility courses and a dog dancing course. As her owner noticed that both dogs became more and more nervous and worked up and that Diego had made no progress whatsoever in his social behavior, she left the school.

In hindsight, she believes that the trainer ignored her constant pleas for individual training focusing on meeting other dogs because the trainer herself was overwhelmed by the situation and didn't know how to solve Diego's problem. She didn't even see that his behavior had in fact seriously deteriorated. In her opinion, Ms Trobisch was the biggest problem, because she was too anxious and insecure with such a big dog.

In early 2002, Ms Trobisch, Diego and Anna paid their first visit to my dog school. I will never forget the first time I met them. A long path leads along a stream to my dog school and from a long way off I saw a tall, slim woman flying along the path, her feet almost lifting off the ground. I was surprised at how she managed to hold the two at all. After she arrived on the training area, I asked her to unleash the two dogs. I wanted to see what the two did when they ran free. But what happened next I had never seen before. The moment the leash was off they ran around like exploding rockets. For an entire 18 minutes they ran at full tilt around the 3,000 square foot area without taking any break worth mention-

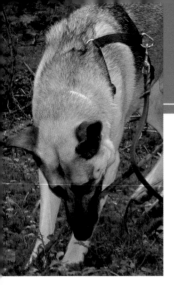

ing. That means that none of the dogs stood for longer than 20 seconds on one spot. Even then, they didn't stand still, but hopped from one leg to the other with a totally wild look on their faces. They only stood still when they wanted to orientate themselves. The moment they discovered another dog on the other side of the fence, they charged over at top speed and crashed into the wire fence, barking, baring their teeth, completely out of their minds. I had never before seen one dog behave so frantically, let alone in a double pack.

After Ms Trobisch had explained the history of the dogs, we went into the consultation room to talk in depth about the living circumstances, stress, feeding, etc. I then found out that, in addition to this stress-inducing training, the dogs spent an hour every day in the garden having the ball thrown to them in an effort to tire them out. In winter, when Ms Trobisch threw snow balls, Diego was so worked up that he bit her hands.

The following anti-stress program was established:

- First, we restructured basic obedience. The most important element was to remove the ball as reward and to calm Diego down enough so that he would accept a treat. This was achieved relatively quickly. It was also important for Diego to work in peace and quiet and away from all other dogs. He was at this time so stressed that he went crazy at the mere sight of another dog, even when it was a long way off. Additionally, he could build up a trusting relationship with me as trainer.

- Ball play was greatly reduced – it was not possible to immediately cut it out altogether. At this point in time, Diego was at the peak of both mental and physical fitness and needed to "wind down" carefully. It could be compared with a marathon runner whose body and psyche is conditioned to running 20 miles a day. If this person were to stop running from one day to another, this would result in physical as well as psychological problems.

- Communicative walking. This entails human and dog really going for walks together. For Ms Trobisch and her dogs this was not the case. Ms Trobisch had been relegated to the status of chauffeur and ball-server. She had to work on the dogs relating to her as a person again. Here she paid more attention to her dogs' eye contact, to which she responded. She got the dogs involved in small activities that they could carry out together, such as balancing on a tree trunk, etc.

- She also had to learn to walk slowly and more calmly. Ms Trobisch walked too quickly, which was carried over to the dogs. The moment she reduced her tempo, she noticed that her dogs also became calmer.

- She was additionally asked to go for walks where there were very few distractions in order to reduce any possible triggering factors. Hour-long rambling or mountain trips were to be avoided in the following weeks.

- We trained her to quiet her voice in order to radiate as much calm as possible, likewise with her body language. It never fails to amaze me how a calm, gentle, but nevertheless poised voice and simplified body language works on the dog. Practically every dog becomes instantly calmer.

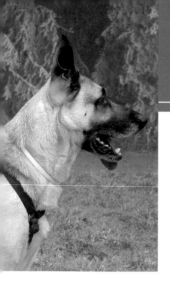

- Both dogs reach a high speed very quickly during play. It is important to give them the opportunity to properly romp around. On the other hand, we did not want to give them the chance to wind each other up. So we developed a concept that worked well for the pair of them. In the mornings both went for a walk on the leash for 15 to 30 minutes. In the afternoons or evenings they went for an hour, whereby they only twice had the opportunity to both run free at the same time in order to have a good run. During the rest of the walk one of the dogs ran free while the other stayed on the leash, swapping over every five minutes. Once in a while the dogs were taken for separate walks.

- We got rid of the head halter and changed both dogs over to harnesses and 10-foot long leather leashes. The harness distributes the pressure over the chest, away from the sensitive neck vertebrae and throat. The handle on the back allows you to hold even large, powerful dogs much better than with a collar. A 10-foot leash gives the dog enough opportunity to go left and right without needing to pull against the leash. It is often the case that a leash that is too short is the reason why dogs pull. If the leash is too short and the dog reaches the end of it after only two or three steps forward, he has no other option than to pull. Many people who are at their wits' end with their leash-tugging dogs, are delighted to see how easy it is when the dog has enough movement to run free.

- A further point of the training involved Ms Trobisch learning how to recognize her dogs' calming signals and how to interpret them in relation to the situation. Likewise she learned how to display them herself if her dogs became anxious or restless.

- The garden was re-arranged slightly. Previously, Diego and Anna were able to run up to the front-facing part of the garden fence and let any passers-by know their presence was unwelcome. They made frequent and loud use of this opportunity, which was neither good for their peace of mind nor for Ms Trobisch or the neighbors. Ms Trobisch made sure that the dogs were only allowed to go into the rear part of the garden in order to bring the circus at the fence to an end.

- Finally we changed the food. Previously both dogs were fed with dry food with a high protein and fat content. Now they eat only wet food with a much lower protein and fat content.

After approximately four weeks of twice-weekly appointments we had got to the point where we could work on the obstacles course. The aim here is not to get the dogs as quickly as possible through the course and it is completely irrelevant which order they do it in.

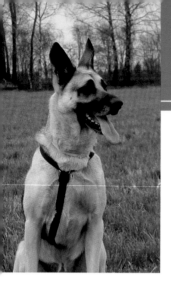

Concentrated slowness is the motto. The dog should get to know and master the obstacles and the various levels of difficulty at his or her own pace. This requires patience, concentration and poise on the part of the human who guides the dog through the training.

Always remember that, if you want your dog to be well balanced and calm, then you must also be well balanced and calm. If you continue to be impatient, hectic, loud and nervous, you cannot be a model of poise and appropriate behavior for your dog!

On top of this it is important for human and dog to really work together through the obstacles. This is the only way to build trust and strengthen the bond.

During basic obedience training and working with obstacles we used an extra tool that we call "the calming pause." This means that the dog is encouraged to rest for a short time during the carrying out of commands such as "sit" and "stay."

A number of issues are important to be aware of here:

- That the dog must know his commands, i.e., he must be aware of what he is expected to do.

- At the beginning the "calming pause" tool would be used only in non-distracting environments. For Diego in particular it was an amazing achievement for him to sit still for even a second. The exercise would never have worked if there had been any distractions, however small.

- Having to carry out a command would never be used as a form of punishment! The dog should never be given the impression that commands are what he is confronted with when his owner is annoyed or when a bad mood is in the air. The golden rule: commands are always good and bring hope of something nice like treats, praise or something enjoyable for the dog. In this way you create positive expectations and concentrated attentiveness.

- The exercise must under no circumstances last too long. For Diego we began with a sit exercise of around five seconds.

- The body language and voice of the person working with the dog is considerably lowered for, as previously mentioned, when you hop around the dog making high-pitched noises, there is NO WAY he can relax. Mood transfer does not just occur from dog to dog but also from human to dog, and vice versa.

- The dog should have already had enough opportunity to satisfy his need for movement. It would make no sense for the dog to begin with exercises like "the calming pause" when he has just arrived at the training ground.

- The "calming pause" tool is never used when the dog feels threatened by another human, dog or animal. It would be unfair to force the dog into a defenseless position.

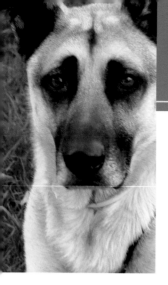

Even at the beginning when Diego could only tolerate the commands that were supposed to calm him down for a few seconds, he made clear progress. After nine individual training sessions we added a further training element into the mix, something we call "changing the association." Among other factors, dogs learn through association. For months, Diego had associated meeting dogs – even the very sight of them – with unpleasantness and had to protect himself by responding with aggression the moment a certain distance was overstepped. When I met Diego this distance was around 600 feet! We had to change the association of seeing another dog to something either neutral or (even better) positive. From the very beginning, I did not share the trainer's and vet's opinion that Diego was dominant towards other male dogs. This dog was only one thing – STRESSED – and to an extent I had never seen before.

As we began the changing the association training, our goal was at some point to get Diego to be able to pass another dog within 6 to 10 feet without flipping out. We achieved this amazingly quickly. Diego understood almost immediately that the other dogs would not come too near and he remained calm so long as he got enough support from his owner. We had, up to this point, only worked with female dogs and, as this had worked wonderfully, we wanted to try it out with males. For this reason, we brought in Chenook, my large male Hovawart, German Shepherd and Collie cross.

Chenook remained completely calm at my side. Diego carried out the familiar training exercises but, as Chenook and I got within 20 feet of him and Ms Trobisch, he froze completely. He stood there with a vacant stare, tail clamped between his spread legs, incapable of reaction – he did not know how to behave and could not cope any more. Of course we immediately put distance between us so that Diego felt better again. I felt really sorry for him but nevertheless it had been a useful experience. Diego did not lunge forward aggressively! He had obviously put aside this behavioral pattern but had still no idea how else he should behave! We could not leave him hanging there at this stage of uncertainty. Ms Trobisch stayed with Diego at a great enough distance to myself and Chenook, rewarding even the tiniest of calming signals that he displayed. When he dared even a glance in our direction, she spoke reassuringly and rewarded him. Additionally, she gave him physical contact by placing herself right next to him. After a few rounds of this we ended our training. Diego slept like a stone in the car and at home for hours on end. This gives you an indication of how exhausting the situation was for him. Indeed it was often not possible to work with Diego for longer than 15 minutes because his concentration deteriorated and so tended more towards regression than progress.

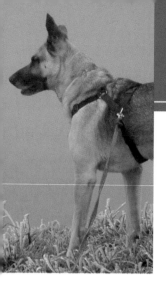

Of course, regression occurred anyway. Distances to other dogs that had been easily managed in previous training sessions suddenly became a problem again. He was no longer able to carry out exercises he had long since mastered – sometimes he seemed to have forgotten them completely. When Ms Trobisch and I talked about events of the preceding days, we often found out what it was that had stressed Diego. And from time to time we had absolutely no idea what was wrong with him. Thankfully these moments were few.

One of the most frustrating times was summer 2002. We had initially separated Anna and Diego for training. Anna had been integrated into a mixed group of dogs (large, small, young, old, male, female) that she visited once a week. She got the opportunity to have peaceful (!) contact with other dogs – which worked well. At the beginning, we had to make sure that Anna did not get too worked up by running around and become rough. But eventually she became more secure and accustomed to being around other dogs.

The next step was for Diego and Anna to go past other dogs together. This exercise had worked wonderfully when each dog did it individually, so we thought it was worth trying them together. A total disaster! Anna (not Diego) wound the pair of them up immediately on seeing the other dog. The same old routine! We seriously considered whether it would be better to separate the dogs and find a new home for Anna – but dismissed the idea because the dogs were devoted to each other and Ms Trobisch was almost in tears at the thought of giving Anna away. Frustrated, we called it quits for the day.

Shortly after, a new problem appeared. After the ball play had been fully scrapped, Diego searched for replacement prey – in the form of joggers, cyclists and so on. The faster something moved the more interested he was in chasing after it.

The consequences for training were:

- Use of a thirty-foot long leash in order to be able to control Diego better.

- Increased practice of the recall command.

- Choice of a wide-open piece of land so that no jogger can suddenly come running around the corner and appear directly in front of Diego.

- Play with the ball again, but only a little!

Incidentally, we also had Diego's thyroid checked out because an illness in this region can also lead to over-reactions. His values were normal.

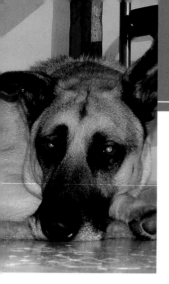

In April, Ms Trobisch decided to have Diego neutered. We had considered this option at length and asked two other competent trainers what they thought. Both met Diego and were also of the opinion that a castration could help to lower his stress levels. After the operation, Diego had a long break from training so that the wounds could heal properly. In June we carried on with the training and discovered that Diego had regressed. Obviously it was still essential for him to have regular training. However, the castration turned out to be the right thing to do as, three to four months after the operation, Diego became much calmer and more well balanced. He was still very energetic, but generally more manageable. After the training had been going on regularly for a while Diego's progress picked up.

In August, Diego was nervous and agitated again. We found out that Ms Trobisch's parents had paid a three-week visit with their Collie puppy, something that was clearly too much for Diego. Nevertheless, it should be seen as an incredible success that Diego had accepted this strange dog into his house at all.

Big success at the end of August! Ms Trobisch rang me full of joy to tell me that Diego had growled at a female dog that wanted to jump into his car. Other dog owners would have probably not been so delighted by this but Ms Trobisch was schooled enough to know what this meant. Diego had kept his nerve and only threatened the female dog, which she immediately reacted to by going away from the car. Earlier he would have gone berserk on her. A very big day in Diego's life – he had learned how to warn.

Further progress followed. Joggers, cyclists and so on are no longer a problem. Diego is much calmer, but still temperamental. He looks for physical contact of his own accord with his owner and wants to cuddle. He even walks much better on the leash now, even if he still pulls and Ms Trobisch's image of the dog walking happily on a loose leash next to her is still only a distant dream. Two or three encounters with other dogs ended peacefully. Once Diego met an entire group of dogs among whom he could move around without any problem. But not all meetings are without their problems. In general there are good and bad days, but the bad days are waning. The training is still going on. Tomorrow I will see him and Ms Trobisch again. We want to try and get him to go for walks with another dog. The chances of this being successful are high. Ms Trobisch says her knees buckle at the prospect of it and hopes that everything will be all right. I am confident. Diego has made so much progress already and is a wonderful dog. He just needs a little more time…

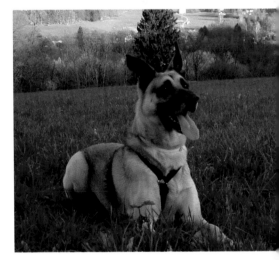

MONA

Mona arrived at her new home at the age of nine weeks. Mr and Mrs Maier had both retired at the age of 60 and wanted to fulfill their long-held dream of owning a dog. Friends of theirs had bred Giant Schnauzers for years and had enthused the Maiers about this breed. From a litter they chose a female puppy that was considered to be the most affectionate and gentle.

Mona was bred in ideal conditions. She lived with her mother and siblings in the house. The litter was bedded down in a room bordering the living room, with a flap allowing constant access to the garden. They had plenty of contact with other dogs, humans and other stimuli without the puppies being overwhelmed. Mona's mother was well-balanced, friendly and quiet and took loving care of her brood.

The Maiers had prepared themselves very well for their new puppy. In addition to lots of information from friends, they also received good advice from a vet, had read plenty of recommended books about puppies and made sure that they were well prepared for what was to come. They placed Mona's basket in their bedroom so that she wouldn't be alone at night. They visited puppy play groups, made sure she came into contact with friends and neighbors' children, made sure she got a well-balanced diet and kept her healthy. Mona developed wonderfully and became a well-balanced and friendly dog. When the Maiers went on holiday, they took Mona with them because they didn't want to give her to strangers or put her in a boarding kennel.

Life with Mona was as wonderful for the Maiers as they dreamed it would be – until Summer 2001. At this time Mona was three. Like many times before, she was playing in the garden with the neighbors' children, when suddenly a child's screams tore through the air, screams which the Maiers immediately knew meant that something was terribly wrong. They ran into the garden and saw one of the children, a little girl, lying on the ground, screaming, her hands covering her face. There was blood everywhere and the other children were crying and running away, but it was still not certain what had happened. Mrs Maier noticed that Mona, panting heavily, was lying under the bushes with a distraught look on her face. At first, it didn't occur to anyone to think that she was the cause of the injury. Only when one of the children told how Mona had bitten Sarah was it clear what the dog had done to the child.

The parents rushed off to the hospital with their child, where Sarah was treated and the extent of the injuries was ascertained. After the initial medical treatment, Sarah had to undergo a number of operations before her face once more resembled that of the nice little girl she was before the incident. Just as bad as the physical injuries were the mental wounds. When she saw a dog in the distance she began to cry and wanted to run away. Sarah's parents then decided to consult a child psychologist who could help their daughter get over the traumatic events of that fateful afternoon.

Back to Mona. Nobody was able to explain why she had bitten. She knew all of the children present for a long time and loved playing with them. She had never before shown even the slightest hint of aggression. Quite the contrary. The alleged innate aggression of the breed was nowhere to be seen in her, leading to her being nicknamed the "little sheep", "snail," and "dreamer."

Together with the other children, the parents and Mona's owners it was possible to work out what had happened. The day in question was a 90 degree scorcher. Mona and the children began to play in the garden at around 2 pm while the Maiers sat in the cool shade of their living room. The parents of one of the children were also sitting in the shade of a neighboring garden, occasionally looking over from time to time. The incident occurred at 3 pm. On being questioned the children and adults said that Mona and the children had been playing the entire time and that Mona had been panting heavily. She tried on a number of occasions to withdraw into the bushes but was always enticed out by one of the children because they wanted to play with her a bit more. When she wouldn't come out anymore, despite all temptations, the children grabbed her by her collar and dragged her out. The moment they let go she fled back into the bushes. When little Sarah then went into the bushes to pull Mona out once more, she growled and bared her teeth. When Sarah then increased the pressure on the collar, Mona bit her. As Sarah was eye to eye with the dog, the bites struck her in the face.

After reconstructing what had happened it became clear that Mona was the least guilty (if at all) party involved in the incident. What was so remarkable was that the service dog handler designated to investigate the incident came to exactly the same conclusion. This was all the more remarkable considering it was the year 2001, when a media frenzy of hate against dogs – and their owners - was sweeping through Germany after in Hamburg a boy was killed by a so-called fighting dog.

Mona's social fitness for people was officially tested and found to be excellent. In the final report it was stated that the dog had been extremely stressed due to physical and mental exhaustion caused by playing for too long in high temperatures and without adult supervision. The dog had no other option, after all attempts to withdraw had failed, than to bite.

Both the Maiers as well as the parents who were in the neighboring gardens were accused – and quite rightly so - of having failed to provide adequate supervision.

Mr and Mrs Maier toyed with the idea of giving Mona away. They both felt that they had failed and were plagued by feelings of guilt. They also believed that a dog that had bitten could not be trusted – a stupid prejudice that is often heard and fortunately easily disprove.

In the meantime, one and a half years down the line, Mona has shown no sign of aggressive behavior.

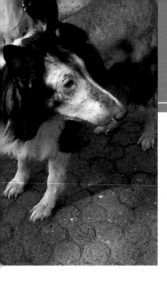

LUCIA

We received a call from Margit Koopmann of the animal rescue organization "Collies in Need" who asked us if we would take care of a female collie which was in a terrible state. She told us it was an emergency and that the dog had been brought to a veterinary clinic by the owner, who was not interested in having the dog examined and treated because it was too expensive. The dog was faced with being euthanized. First, this was what the owner wanted, second there was nobody who was willing to pay for the treatment and, third, it was questionable whether treatment was worthwhile because the future of the dog was not clear. One of the vets asked the organization for help because she felt sorry for the dog and also saw no reason to have the dog put down. Lucia had heavy hair loss and skin lesions and was not nice to look at, which reduced her chances of being found a home. Yet, this could be dealt with the moment they found out what was actually wrong with her. Blood and skin tests had been carried out but nothing had been found and so they were none the wiser about the cause. She was infested with fleas but the fleas alone could not explain the desolate state she was in. Some suspected that her condition could be partly stress-induced and of psychological nature because she was treated very unlovingly by her owner and was totally exhausted.

We were told that she had been kept in a yard and was not allowed into the house. She was not provided with any form of accommodation such as a hut or kennel. She was given only poor-quality food and was badly treated by her owner.

We agreed to take her and she arrived the next day. Indeed, she looked terrible. There was hardly anything left of her coat, she was practically naked. Her skin was covered in scabs and heavily puffed up, in some areas bleeding and weeping. Her face was the most affected region. She stank so badly that only the strongest of stomachs could face being in the same room as her for any length of time without gagging. She was suitably exhausted by the long car journey and the various strange people, but didn't appear to be psychologically worse for wear. In fact we were even surprised at just how good she seemed, considering the circumstances.

One of our employees at the time, Barbara Gleixner, offered to take Lucia (that was what we called her) and look after her until she was well enough to be found a new home. Barbara lived at that time with her four dogs and seven cats in a small house in the middle of the forest. The house stood in a clearing and deer came up to her front door even in the middle of the day. No neighbors, no roads, no noise, and the post box was two kilometres away, which meant that even the postman didn't come to the door. Pure peace, an absolute idyll, a tiny paradise, and just the right thing for Lucia. She thought so too! She fitted in immediately in this little community and above all did one thing – sleep. She slept and slept and slept. Only after a few days did she begin to get involved with the other four-legged members of the household and quickly made friends.

During this time Lucia was once again thoroughly examined by our vet and a slight metabolic disorder was discovered. It was however not so bad that it could sufficiently explain Lucia's desolate physical condition. Barbara decided to detoxify Lucia and prepared a few homeopathic remedies for her.

I saw Lucia three days after her arrival. She still looked terrible and stank intensively but she did not give the impression of being afraid of what was coming next, as so many other animals that have been through such bad times do. Lucia seemed to trust us totally, which really touched me, as her previous experience of humans left a lot to be desired. She was friendly and open, seemed however very exhausted, reacted nervously to loud or sudden noises and moved noticeably slowly - not exactly in a timid and careful way, but more like someone for whom everything is just too much.

After only one week the skin had dried out and the bloody patches scabbed over and then fell off. A short time later, the first tufts of fluff appeared on the previously bald patches of skin. We were over the moon about this. The stench gradually faded and disappeared completely after three or four weeks. With time the hair grew back.

It gradually became time for Lucia to find a new home. One of the dog school trainees, Frank Bressel, was my favorite choice. He is a quiet and well-balanced man with a big heart for all dogs in the world. And indeed Lucia ended up with him and his family. Barbara and I were happy because it could not have been better than this: wonderful people who knew all about dogs, a house with garden and four-legged house member, Mandy, the Bernese Mountain Dog. We were also happy that we had the chance to see Lucia from time to time during Franks' regular visits, so contact was not completely broken off.

We firmly believe that stress was the main cause of Lucia's bad physical state. Our vet confirmed this belief because the metabolic disorder she had (the only thing that could be found wrong with her) disappeared of its own accord after Lucia had found peace and her mental balance once again. The anti-stress program involved:

- Showing her love and security
- Giving her enough places to withdraw to, to rest and sleep
- Giving her a life suitable for a dog - contact with other dogs, friendly cats and people
- Walks in the fresh air, and
- A healthy diet

That was all. Lucia is completely healthy again.

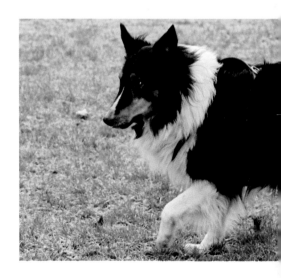

WOLFGANG AND BERND

Wolfgang is a handsome, male Bernese Mountain Dog, who came as a puppy to the Pleuger family, where he was to spend his whole life. Wolfgang came to the family when the Pleugers' son was eight and the daughter was six. The idea was that the children would grow up with a pet and, as the postman's female dog had just had puppies, Wolfgang was chosen. Over time, the children grew up and Wolfgang turned into an 11 year old gentlman, a good age for such a large dog. The Pleugers looked back on the many wonderful memories of the years that seemed to have shot by and felt very melancholic about the thought that he wouldn't be with them for much longer. It was difficult for him to stand up because he had a hip problem and his joints were not as smooth as they once were and showed signs of wear. On warm days he had problems with his circulation and was prescribed with drops that he had to take every morning. A friend of the family advised them to get a new dog before Wolfgang died, preferably a puppy, as Wolfgang could help to raise him and he would take on all of the wonderful characteristics that the Pleugers liked in Wolfgang so much. So, they got Bernd. As the Pleugers had had such good experience with Bernese Mountain Dogs, they opted for a dog of the same breed, went to a breeder that had been recommended to them and chose the strongest and most lively puppy in the litter. Delighted with the little tyke, they returned home and introduced him to Wolfgang. To their disappointment, he showed no interest in the new addition to the family. He sniffed him thoroughly, then lay down in his basket with a sigh and slept.

Over the next few days, a mass of new visitors - friends and acquaintances – were called by the Pleugers and came to see Bernd. In contrast to Wolfgang, they were beyond themselves with joy over the little, clumsy pup, who seemed to have great difficulty dealing with his huge paws. Wolfgang seemed to be happy to retreat to his basket and sleep or doze. The fuss was apparently just too much for him.

Thankfully, the attraction wore off and the visits became less frequent and it became quieter in the house and Bernd became bored. As could only be expected of a puppy, he wanted to play. He was constantly out and about to discover new things in the house and garden. In the evening he seemed to be possessed by the typical puppy "five minutes", in which he would race throughout the house barking and sweep away everything in his path. If he got close to Wolfgang or tried to entice him to play, he was growled at. The Pleugers never thought this would happen. They couldn't understand why Wolfgang got so annoyed and thought he was jealous because Bernd attracted so much attention. They told Wolfgang off for his behavior and reminded him that Bernd had a "puppy license" and so he had to be nice to him. They had read this in a book in which it also said that male dogs in particular were very loving and patient with youngsters.

When the Pleugers went for a walk with Wolfgang and Bernd, Bernd at first tried to get Wolfgang to play. At the best, Wolfgang's response was clear growls. If Bernd didn't immediately go away, Wolfgang snapped at him. Bernd yelped and toddled off. All of his friendly approaches were turned down by the older fellow, which was not a nice experience for a puppy. Once, Bernd tried to snuggle next to Wolfgang in his basket. If the Pleugers hadn't pulled Bernd away quickly enough, it could have turned nasty, as Wolfgang had bared his teeth to the point of almost biting. Soon, the situation had escalated between the young and the old dogs to such an extent that Bernd sneaked through the house and garden when Wolfgang was nearby. And Wolfgang himself tried to stay out of Bernd's way. Another time the Pleugers were going for a walk with both dogs when Bernd bumped into Wolfgang's flank while enthusiastically chasing a butterfly. Wolfgang reacted by burying Bernd under him with thunderous growling and bared teeth. The Pleugers separated the two dogs. Nothing much had happened, Bernd had a few scratches and was visibly shocked, but it had become clear that the situation between the two had got very bad indeed. Wolfgang had changed completely. Before he was quiet and friendly to other dogs and humans. Now he was constantly annoyed, had even started to growl at other dogs, and even at the Pleugers themselves. This had not happened once over the previous years and the thought occurred to them that he might have had some sort of tumor. They made an appointment at my dog school in order to get some advice.

After I listened to the complete story, we talked about the situation. I explained to the Pleugers that it cannot be assumed that every adult dog is fond of puppies. The much quoted – and untrue – so-called "puppy license" does not exist. It is correct to state that canine tolerance of puppies is greater than toward adult dogs but that does not mean that a puppy can and is allowed to do what he wants without being disciplined. If that were the case, then the puppy would not need to be educated by the older dog.

Wolfgang's behavior led us to conclude that he was irritated and stressed by the puppy's presence. This explained his annoyance and aggression. A brain tumor, the diagnostic ghoul of veterinary medicine constantly used as an explanation for all manner of unusual behavior when nothing else seemed to fit, could almost certainly be ruled out. Firstly, the chances that a dog has a brain tumor are statistically slight. Further, Wolfgang showed none of the symptoms that normally accompany a brain tumor, such as diminished sensory functionality, epileptic fits, disorientation, co-ordination problems, etc.

However, Wolfgang was indeed sick. The age-related complaints mentioned previously were causing him pain. He needed peace. I explained to the Pleugers that they had to accept that Wolfgang was no longer just the "old man", but was just old. He wasn't as easy-going and well-balanced as he once was. In humans, the ability to compensate for stress decreases as we get older, and this is the same in dogs. Bernd's presence was just too much for Wolfgang and the friend's advice to get a puppy was totally wrong.

They also had to consider that the conditions in which Bernd was growing up were no fun for him, either. Instead of messing around and being as silly as he wanted, he crept around the house with his tail between his legs. In the meantime, he stopped playing completely the moment he saw Wolfgang and lay on his blanket as quiet as a church mouse, or left the room. Worse still was that this behavior was being played out on other dogs he met during walks and he appeared timid and anxious in their presence. This was not a good development and had to be changed as quickly as possible. I urged the Pleugers to find Bernd a new home. Of course, tears flowed but they finally decided to find a new home for Bernd, in which he could grow up without problems. In fact, he ended up staying in the family, as Mrs Pleuger's sister took him after hearing he was to be given away. Everybody breathed a sigh of relief, Wolfgang probably the most. He recovered fairly quickly and became as friendly and well-balanced as he had always been. Bernd is now one year old and occasionally Mrs Pleuger, her sister, Wolfgang and Bernd go for walks together. The dogs get on but Mrs Pleuger has the feeling that Wolfgang is always happy when he can go home with her. And Mrs Pleuger's sister told me recently that Bernd is always happy when the "old guy" comes home and the two can have some real fun together, throwing sticks, barking loudly and running wildly through streams and over the fields.

STRESS REDUCING SOLUTIONS

These cases show that there is no magic remedy for an anti-stress program. The solutions are as various as the symptoms of the individual dogs themselves. Nevertheless, there are a few points that can be generally followed in order to keep the dog's stress levels as low as possible.

- Make sure that your dog has sufficient periods of rest during the day and make sure he is not disturbed.

- When you have visitors, go to a cafe, visit friends or do any other activity, look at your dog's calming signals or behavior to see if everything is getting too much for him. Think also about whether it makes sense to take the dog everywhere you go. Sometimes we think it is nice for our dog to go shopping with us, or go to work, or to visit friends and so on. And sometimes that is the case. But keep in mind that your dog can have too much of a good thing.

- If you are considering getting another dog, a cat or another pet, think about how you believe your dog will be able to deal with the new addition to the family. When choosing the new dog, you should, under all circumstances, let your current dog have a role in deciding. As could be seen in the case of Wolfgang and Bernd, not every dog is happy about the new four-legged family member. On the other hand, you should not assume that two dogs do not like each other just because they don't play with each other in the first ten minutes. Humans also need time to get to know each other before we decide whether we want to be friends.

- Your dog should have the opportunity to use his instinctive behaviors (naturally, only as far as this is possible, because you of course cannot allow him to chase wild animals). But you can give him the opportunity to use the fantastic abilities of his nose by giving him searching exercises. You will experience how enthusiastically your dog co-operates, and slumbers away in his basket afterwards.

- Give your dog the time to find out about what is around him. This is particularly important when you visit a new place, whether it is the training area of a dog school or a friend's apartment that is unfamiliar to him. Let him explore the new surroundings in peace. Let him look around, sniff and walk through the room if he wants. Only when he has got to know this new place will he feel safe and happy there. Offer him a familiar blanket or jacket to lie on without commanding him to do so.

Think about how you would behave if you arrived in a strange place. Imagine, for instance, you attend a seminar. You drive to the venue and are already having thoughts about whether you will find the way, whether everything is all right with the reservation and what the people will be like. You notice that you are slightly anxious and nervous. Eventually you arrive and enter the room where the event will take place. A few people have already arrived, but you do not know anyone. What do you do? Most likely you take a short look around to explore the surroundings. Maybe you contemplate where your room and the restrooms might be. If there are stands with brochures, books or items for sale, you take a look around. With a bit of luck, you strike up a conversation with someone and you start to feel more secure. When you then find a chair with your name on it you feel better because you now know where you're supposed to sit and that you are actually expected. The initial tension disappears. On the following seminar days the surroundings become more familiar to you and you take your chair without further thought. The situation has been clarified and you are relaxed.

- Should you and your dog attend a seminar or go to a restaurant or anything similar, let him decide whether he wants to sit, lie down or stand. In this way, it is possible for your dog to find the most comfortable spot possible. Don't insist on him constantly carrying out the "sit" and "down" command. See how much you demand of your dog – often without thinking about it – and "pull the brake" if it's getting too much for him. If your dog behaves restlessly, tries to get out of your way or often looks out the door, this is a sure sign that everything is getting too much for him.

- Your dog should have the chance to relieve himself when he needs to.

- Periods of excitement should be followed by periods of rest.

- When your dog is stressed because he is afraid of something, make sure that you keep a good distance between him and the creature or object that is causing the fear. Depending on the circumstances, this distance could be large. In all cases give your dog the opportunity to keep the scary "something" in his sights. Imagine you had to be in a room with something you were afraid of. Wouldn't you want to make sure you kept a good eye on it? Wouldn't it be important for you to know where it was? Wouldn't you want to know if it was heading toward you and, if so, how fast?

- Create rituals that give your dog the security of knowing what is coming next.

- Make sure you hold the leash loosely. A tensed and short leash causes your dog additional stress. He doesn't just feel the unpleasant pull but has at the same time the feeling that he can't get away. Also, for almost all dogs, wearing a harness is much more pleasant than a collar.

- Show your dog that YOU have the situation under control and will protect him where necessary. Give him the feeling that you are there for him and, if he is scared, he can hide behind you. Help him out of situations that overwhelm him. In other words, behave in the same way as good parents do towards their children. Of course, you shouldn't be over-protective but, if he has learned that he can rely on you in difficult moments, this will give him a lot of security.

- Speak to your dog in a calm, gentle and friendly voice.

- Get him gradually accustomed to situations that often occur in daily life, such as car trips, visits to the vet, being taken to the office, etc. But make sure that your well-intentioned efforts don't end up overwhelming your dog.

- The golden rule is: less is more. If you are not sure whether something is too much for your dog or not, stop training or get away from the situation.

- Create the opportunity for success and reward. You are responsible for planning situations in such a way that your dog can go from one small success to another.

- When you play with your dog, make sure you don't get him worked up. Quieter activities such as exploring a piece of land together, or searching games where your dog has to use his nose, are much more suitable than the hectic chase games.

- Don't expect too much at once from either your dog or yourself!

ACKNOWLEDGMENTS

Our special thanks go out to all of the dogs that we have learned from during training and endless hours of observation, and Turid Rugaas, who made us think so much about everything to do with dogs and brought the topic of stress to our attention, and together we developed the idea for this book.

We would like to additionally thank our husbands for their understanding when we were yet again up to our necks in it in the office, were incommunicado and who had to deal with the telephone and the dogs.

We would like to thank Anke Rasch-Sahle for her patient proof-reading of the manuscript.

Martina Scholz & Clarissa von Reinhardt

RECOMMENDED READING/ SOURCES

Turid Rugaas, On Talking Terms With Dogs: Calming Signals 2nd Ed.
Dogwise Publishing, 2006

G.P. Moberg and J.A. Mench, The biology of animal stress –
basic principles and implications for animal welfare
CABI Publishing

Anders Hallgren, Hundeprobleme – Problemhunde
Dog problems – problem dogs)
Oertel + Spörer, Reutlingen 1993, ISBN 3-88627-127-7

Raymond and Lorna Coppinger, Dogs: A New Understanding of Canine Origin,
Behavior, and Evolution. University of Chicago Press, 2001

B.W. Knol, Behavior problems in dogs: a review of problems,
diagnosis, therapeutic measures and results in 133 patients,
In: Veterinary Quarterly 1987, No. 9, page 226 – 234

B.W. Knol, Influence of stress on the motivation for agonistic behavior in the male
dog, 1988

Dietmar Juli and Maren Engelbrecht-Greve, Stressverhalten ändern lernen –
Programm zum Abbau psychosomatischer Krankheitsrisiken,
Rowohlt Taschenbuch Verlag, Reinbek 1991, ISBN 3-499-17193-7

Brockhaus Encyclopedia in 24 volumes
F.A. Brockhaus Verlag Mannheim, 19th edition, ISBN 3-7653-1100-6

Pschyrembel Klinisches Wörterbuch (clinical dictionary),
Walter de Gruyter GmbH, Berlin, 255th Edition, ISBN 3-1100-7916-X

INDEX

From Dogwise Publishing, www.dogwise.com, 1-800-776-2665

BEHAVIOR & TRAINING

ABC's of Behav'r Shaping; Fundmtls of Train'g; Proactive Behav'r Mgmt, DVD. Ted Turner
Aggression In Dogs: Practical Mgmt, Prevention & Behaviour Modification. Brenda Aloff
Am I Safe? DVD. Sarah Kalnajs
Behavior Problems in Dogs, 3rd ed. William Campbell
Brenda Aloff's Fundamentals: Foundation Training for Every Dog, DVD. Brenda Aloff
Bringing Light to Shadow. A Dog Trainer's Diary. Pam Dennison
Canine Body Language. A Photographic Gd to the Native Language of Dogs. Brenda Aloff
Clicked Retriever. Lana Mitchell
Dog Behavior Problems: The Counselor's Handbook. William Campbell
Dog Friendly Gardens, Garden Friendly Dogs. Cheryl Smith
Dog Language, An Encyclopedia of Canine Behavior. Roger Abrantes
Evolution of Canine Social Behavior, 2nd ed. Roger Abrantes
Give Them a Scalpel and They Will Dissect a Kiss, DVD. Ian Dunbar
Guide To Professional Dog Walking And Home Boarding. Dianne Eibner
Language of Dogs, DVD. Sarah Kalnajs
Mastering Variable Surface Tracking, Component Tracking (2 bk set). Ed Presnall
My Dog Pulls. What Do I Do? Turid Rugaas
New Knowledge of Dog Behavior (reprint). Clarence Pfaffenberger
On Talking Terms with Dogs: Calming Signals, 2nd edition. Turid Rugaas
On Talking Terms with Dogs: What Your Dog Tells You, DVD. Turid Rugaas
Positive Perspectives: Love Your Dog, Train Your Dog. Pat Miller
Predation and Family Dogs, DVD. Jean Donaldson
Really Reliable Recall. Train Your Dog to Come When Called, DVD. Leslie Nelson
Right on Target. Taking Dog Training to a New Level. Mandy Book & Cheryl Smith
Stress in Dogs. Martina Scholz & Clarissa von Reinhardt
The Dog Trainer's Resource: The APDT Chronicle of the Dog Collection. Mychelle Blake (*ed*)
Therapy Dogs: Training Your Dog To Reach Others. Kathy Diamond Davis
Training Dogs, A Manual (reprint). Konrad Most
Training the Disaster Search Dog. Shirley Hammond
Try Tracking: The Puppy Tracking Primer. Carolyn Krause
When Pigs Fly. Train Your Impossible Dog. Jane Killion
Winning Team. A Guidebook for Junior Showmanship. Gail Haynes
Working Dogs (reprint). Elliot Humphrey & Lucien Warner

HEALTH & ANATOMY, SHOWING

An Eye for a Dog. Illustrated Guide to Judging Purebred Dogs. Robert Cole
Annie On Dogs! Ann Rogers Clark
Canine Cineradiography DVD. Rachel Page Elliott
Canine Massage: A Complete Reference Manual. Jean-Pierre Hourdebaigt
Canine Terminology (reprint). Harold Spira
Dog In Action (reprint). Macdowell Lyon
Dogsteps DVD. Rachel Page Elliott
Performance Dog Nutrition: Optimize Performance With Nutrition. Jocelynn Jacobs
Puppy Intensive Care: A Breeder's Guide To Care Of Newborn Puppies. Myra Savant Harris
Raw Dog Food: Make It Easy for You and Your Dog. Carina MacDonald
Raw Meaty Bones. Tom Lonsdale
Shock to the System. The Facts About Animal Vaccination... Catherine O'Driscoll
The History and Management of the Mastiff. Elizabeth Baxter & Pat Hoffman
Work Wonders. Feed Your Dog Raw Meaty Bones. Tom Lonsdale
Whelping Healthy Puppies, DVD. Sylvia Smart